CW00816130

Disclaimer:

The contents of this book are for general information purposes only and do not establish the granting of medical advice nor the practice of medicine. No doctor-patient relationship is formed directly or in-directly. The contents of this book are not a substitute for the medical advice from your own healthcare professionals. There are no attempts to diagnosis nor treat readers with this information. Instead, it is intended to educate readers while bringing more context and supplementary information to both the reader and their healthcare professionals. The author is not responsible for any misuse of the contents of this book.

TAKE A LOAD OFF

Game Changing Injections for Weight Loss

JONATHAN SCHMIDT, MD

LUCIDBOOKS

Take a Load Off: Game Changing Injections for Weight Loss

Published by Lucid Books in Houston, TX
www.LucidBooks.com

Photo Credit: Bridget Cicchillo

ISBN: 978-1-63296-675-9 (paperback)
ISBN: 978-1-63296-676-6 (hardback)
eISBN: 978-1-63296-677-3

Special Sales: Most Lucid Books titles are available in special quantity discounts. Custom imprinting or excerpting can also be done to fit special needs. Contact Lucid Books at Info@LucidBooks.com

CONTENTS

FOREWORD

Weight has been a touchy or taboo subject in our society for as long as I can remember. It's considered impolite and insulting to ask someone their actual weight. It's considered insulting to comment on a person's eating habits regardless of whether they are too heavy or too skinny. I'm not sure why that is, but it is the world we live in. Other traits are not like that . . . hair color, height, and strength are all personal characteristics that we feel comfortable commenting on with others. But when it comes to weight or behaviors related to weight, the topic is strictly off limits. As a physician of thirteen years, I delicately ask all my patients about their weight during their annual physical. It's not really a surprise that just about every one of my patients wants to lose weight. Some want to lose fifty pounds, but even most people who appear to be average or healthy weight tell me they want to lose five or ten pounds. Weight, and more specifically weight loss, is on the mind of just about everyone I talk with.

For better or worse, we are all thinking about our weight, but most of us aren't acting on a concrete plan to do anything to change it. Lots of technology is available to help us analyze our body and body composition, so we know how much body fat and muscle mass we have. We have apps on our phones that help us track calories; some even make it as simple as just scanning the barcode on the packaging of whatever you are about to put in your mouth. Humans have never had greater access to an abundance of knowledge and resources to help us be successful at controlling our weight. Yet, year after year, my patients keep telling me the same thing: they want to lose weight despite seeing their weight slowly creeping up when they step on the scale at my office each year.

I'm no different than my patients though. I've struggled with my weight over the years as well. First, I wanted to lose five pounds; then it was ten pounds. As I saw larger and larger numbers on the scale, my goals got bigger and bigger. I would try to lose weight for a few weeks or months with moderate success, but it never lasted. By the time I was thirty-nine years old, I was overweight. I was borderline for obesity and on three prescription medications to control my blood pressure and cholesterol. But rather than focusing on making significant healthy changes, I made excuses for myself. Doing the hard work of changing my lifestyle wasn't an option that could reasonably be done. I was exhausted, I was too busy, work was too demanding . . . I needed to enjoy life . . . it's only one cookie . . . let's have dessert three times this week. The list goes on and on; I could convince myself of anything. I was letting the excess weight negatively affect my physical and mental health without even realizing it. I slowly accepted the weight gain even as I promised myself that I wouldn't let the number on the scale go up anymore. But I didn't hold myself accountable when I broke those promises. I'm a physician, and I know full well the harms that come with being overweight or obese, but even that wasn't enough to motivate me to change my habits and do something about my weight.

I can only imagine that my patients were doing the same thing I was doing to myself. They were self-justifying their actions because after all, they were busy, the kids had sports to get to, there wasn't time to make a healthy dinner, they were on vacation, or it was somebody's birthday to celebrate (and it would be rude not to have a piece of cake). What my patients wanted to do and what I needed to do was to make significant healthy lifestyle changes. Lifestyle changes are exactly what they sound like. They are meaningful changes in the way we live our lives day to day. They are not quick fix gimmicks that might work for a short time. Instead, they are changes that we commit to keep doing for the rest of our lives. Lifestyle changes are fundamental changes to our lives whereby we admit we were on the wrong path, change direction, and plot a new path forward.

The problem is that lifestyle changes are hard to make. They aren't fun to make either. Old habits die hard, and food habits are at the core of how we live our lives. This might come from the fact that food is so vital for our survival. But it also comes from the way our society places expectations and norms on us. Society literally puts pressure on us to put food in our mouths. Don't believe me? Think about how we interact with others. When was the last time you met socially with someone, and food wasn't around? We live in a time when food is more abundant than ever. From a historical perspective, it is an unusual privilege that we all take for granted, and most of us haven't adapted well to readily available food. Our society has pressured us into overeating and constantly eating.

For years I've been pushing my patients and myself to make these lifestyle changes—eat a healthier diet, exercise more, focus on their health, get better quality sleep. I know from my medical education the huge impact these healthy changes can have on our lives. That's why I preached them year after year to all my patients. But I couldn't convince or motivate myself (or any of my patients) to accomplish these changes. I was slowly watching patient after patient fall into a downward spiral of gaining a pound or two (or four!) every year. I was watching myself struggle with this downward spiral as well. Yet I couldn't find a way out of it despite my best efforts.

All that changed in the fall of 2022. What I thought was too good to be true became reality with the release of a superior GLP-1 medication (tirzepatide, brand names: Mounjaro and Zepbound). I witnessed a few patients make significant transformations. Some lost twenty to thirty pounds in a matter of months. These were patients who had spent the previous decade failing in their efforts to make any meaningful healthy lifestyle changes.

After celebrating multiple patients' success with weight loss, I decided to try it for myself. I still had my doubts, but I decided my long-term health was at stake, so I undertook the same steps that I advised for my patients. It didn't take long to see results and gain that same motivation to modify my lifestyle. Surprisingly, it was relatively easy. I started living my life as an individual who had a normal healthy weight, and I noticed both physical and mental improvements. It felt like we had finally turned a corner in medicine, and I was excited to help my patients make these drastic lifestyle changes with ease.

That's what I want to do here in *Take a Load Off*. I want to provide the framework for how several of my patients and I accomplished something that we've struggled with for so long. I'll share my story and talk about some of the pitfalls with our current thought process as a medical community. I'm not proposing that everyone should do this, but it worked for me and many of my patients, so I needed to share it with others. There is no promise that it will work for you. The method I'll be describing is new, and we don't know everything about it yet. But I can see the potential for us at a societal level and at an individual level to be able to live a skinnier, healthier life if we want to.

I am so passionate about this topic that I have developed a coaching course to help motivated individuals maintain their weight loss after using GLP-1 medications. If you find yourself identifying with the message in this book, I would love to coach you through your weight-loss journey. Go to my website (www.DirectMDCoach.com) to find out more about that opportunity. For once, something that seems too good to be true, might actually be true. It's an exciting time to be alive!

Chapter 1

DIET AND EXERCISE ARE FAILING

We have all heard the age-old advice that to lose weight, you just need to eat less and move more. Our own personal experience, however, tells us it is so much more complicated than a simple formula of calories in versus calories out that equals our body weight. Our bodies are complex and designed to maintain weight rather than lose weight. Long ago, weight loss was not something anyone would want. Efficiently absorbing calories and saving every single calorie was the key for survival when we didn't know where our next meal was coming from . . . or what it would be. Weight loss is not a natural process, and it is very difficult to accomplish. Therefore, losing weight has become something for which most adults strive but rarely accomplish. In my own practice, I've found that most patients want to lose weight but few are successful.

For years I told patients that they need to do 150 minutes of exercise per week and eat a heart-healthy diet. That's good advice. Everyone should strive to be active in their day-to-day lives and watch their diets. The problem is that our culture is working against us. As a society, we have moved into more sedentary jobs that involve hours of physical inactivity. Sure, a standing desk will help and so will taking breaks to walk around, but our bodies were designed for much more activity than that. I've also concluded that an hour of exercise after work doesn't cancel out the harm that eight hours of staring at a computer screen and not moving does to our bodies and our metabolism. Even our leisure activities are shifting to more sedentary activities. Walks turn into evenings on the couch watching TV. Playing with the dog turns into scrolling through social media. Cooking a healthy meal turns into going out to restaurants.

Exercising is great and provides wonderful benefits, so I encourage my patients to get ample activity each day. In fact, movement throughout your entire life is the key to having a happy, independent retirement on your own terms. Our lives are busy though, and most of us are sleep-deprived. Exercise is often the first thing to get cut from our daily schedule because it is not fun—it's hard work. We falsely believe we can skip a day before getting right back into exercising the next day. In reality, skipping one day just makes it easier to skip another day, and then another . . . and then a week goes by when you didn't exercise at all. After skipping one week, it becomes pretty easy to justify that one week didn't make that big of a difference and before you know it, you haven't worked out in a month and have no plans to start again. That is exactly why most New Year's resolutions fail by February. Schedules are busy, kids are demanding, and work always has one more thing to be accomplished. We all have excuses and unfortunately, we are experts at convincing ourselves that our excuses are good ones. Furthermore, we believe our own lie when we say that we will only take a week off from exercising; in reality, it will be a lot longer before we even consider increasing our activity level again.

The typical American diet consists of food that is loaded with salt and preservatives that aren't doing anyone any good. Our culture is working against us here too. When we socialize with others, food is usually involved. In fact, it can be socially awkward to **not** have food when you are out with others. Portion sizes are out of control at restaurants, training us and our bodies to consume more calories than we need. So, when patients tell me that they don't eat much, I realize that their standards are skewed drastically. Overeating calorie dense food is a double whammy that results in more weight gain despite our efforts to reduce the volume of food we take in. The problem is that we look around and see that "everyone else" is eating this way, so we think it is normal. That leads us to miss the opportunity for improvement that is literally sitting right in front of us.

A 2,000-calorie diet is a great idea on paper. In practice, though, this becomes difficult to accurately achieve unless you are working with a dietitian daily. Patients are notorious for underestimating the number of calories in their food and knowing how big a serving size is. Therefore, they take in multiple servings and end up consuming many more calories than they anticipate. They tend to forget how much they eat over the course of the day and end up thinking that they have eaten very little when in reality, they consumed a lot more calories than needed. Our culture is working against us again by advertising so-called "low calorie" options, which are only low calorie because the serving size is so small that no one is likely to stop eating after one "serving."

Furthermore, tracking calories is complicated by the way the FDA defines the term *calorie*. I am convinced that "zero-calorie" food and drinks that utilize synthetic or artificial sugars are just a marketing gimmick. A zero-calorie soda with artificial sweetener might not be classified as having any calories, but your body uses those zero-calorie, artificially sweetened snacks or drinks as true calories. Moreover, artificial sweeteners cause food to leave your stomach quicker than it otherwise would, which makes it harder to achieve that full feeling. That only adds to the overeating problem because we all want to eat a meal and have our hunger go away.

Intermittent fasting is a breakthrough which has gained popularity. With intermittent fasting, you consume all your calories in an eight-hour window each day and spend the other sixteen hours not taking in any calories. This is a novel idea; this way you don't spend the entire day putting calories in your mouth. Intermittent fasting has a host of benefits that cannot be ignored, and patients who can commit to this pattern of food intake achieve some amazing results. However, taken to the extreme, intermittent fasting can result in your body becoming acidotic, which the medical community calls ketosis. This can be beneficial because ketosis occurs when the body preferentially burn fat for energy instead of sugar, which is why the Keto diet became prevalent. Who wouldn't want to have their body burn extra fat? Both intermittent fasting and the Keto diet offer plenty of benefits and have done a world of good for lots of people. However, I have witnessed patients fail with these because of the marketing gimmicks and social pressures we just discussed.

But my big issue with intermittent fasting and the Keto diet is that the general population views them as diets. And I hate diets. The term *diet* implies that it has a start and end time. Most people have enough willpower to persevere through a week, a month, or several months of self-control and hardship. But that is **not** the right attitude to have at all. We need to think in terms of lifestyle changes—changes that will stay with us for the rest of our lives. Almost everyone I have helped through a Keto diet or intermittent fasting has fallen off course eventually because life gets in the way. It is only possible to white-knuckle or force yourself to do something through sheer willpower for so long before you lose focus and energy.

Lifestyle changes are the key to success. But with our culture working against us on every front, we are set up for failure. Lifestyle changes are hard; we are creatures of habit, and changing our habits is one of the most difficult things we can try to do.

This isn't just a struggle I have helped patients with; it's a struggle that I have lived with for most of my life as well. I'm a doctor; I know what needs to be done. I watch patients succeed and fail with trying to lose weight; I know what works and what doesn't, and I know how we are all so good at manipulating ourselves to believe our excuses. Despite having a front row seat to numerous patients' lives as they struggle with weight loss, I was unable to break through the same cycles to succeed with weight loss or even maintain a steady weight. I watched the numbers on my scale creep up day after day, week after week even as I was tracking my labs and my body composition. I tried to justify to myself that I could accomplish this on my own because, after all, I was giving advice to others about how to be successful with weight management. How could I **not** do this myself? But I failed, and I failed miserably. My dress shirts always felt tight; my pants became shorter as they had to be adjusted higher and higher to accommodate my growing waistline.

The necessary changes were obvious to me and others, but I continued to utilize food as a reward and a comfort while succumbing to the culture around me. I ended up on a cholesterol lowering medication and two blood pressure medications before I turned forty. How could this happen to me? I was doing intermittent fasting . . . most days . . . actually, just on days when I had gotten a good night's sleep. But how often did that happen? I was snoring more and sleeping worse as my weight crept up. The ball was moving in the wrong direction, and it seemed like there was no way to stop it, let alone slow it down. The average American gains four pounds a year . . . that's forty pounds in a decade, and I was more than on track to make that stat a reality in my life. I had seasons when I worked hard and lost weight, but like my patients, those seasons would come to an end, and I would end up heavier than before. It was downright frustrating, but I couldn't find a better solution despite my years of education and training.

KEY POINTS

- ☞ Exercise is important, but with every passing year, it becomes harder to lose weight with exercise alone.
- ☞ Dietary changes are better for weight loss.
  - › Tracking calories is complicated and gets messy quickly.
  - › Fad diets aren't beneficial.
- ☞ Lifestyle modifications and changes are the key to long-term success with weight loss.

Chapter 2

MEDICATIONS HAVE A
BAD TRACK RECORD

Appetite suppressants sound like a wonderful idea; most overweight individuals want to feel hungry less often. Many say that they feel chained to their hunger, and they live much of their lives around that sensation. And if they didn't feel hungry all the time, they would put less food in their mouths, which would lead to weight loss. This all seems perfect in theory, but in practice, it just isn't as clean and simple as this, so it doesn't work out. That's because emotional eating is very real, and often emotions are the cause of most of the calories we take in. Even if we don't think of ourselves as emotional eaters, most of the food we eat has an emotional component to it. The average overweight person takes in more calories after six in the evening than they take in before six.

Modern targeted marketing pushes food at all our senses in every form of media we come across. It is easy for us to consume large quantities of calorie-dense food in a short time. Calorie-dense foods, such as desserts, release the neurohormone dopamine in our brains, which we perceive as a reward. And predictably, we start to crave that sensation because calorie-dense foods make us feel better by releasing dopamine. Once again, the culture hinders our attempts at weight loss because desserts are all around us, making it harder to say no to these sweet treats.

Fen-Phen was the poster child for medical weight loss marketed in the early '90s. Fen-Phen was advertised as a diet pill that would suppress the appetite while stimulating your metabolism. It was advertised as a win-win. Fen-Phen used a two-pronged strategy for weight loss by suppressing your appetite *and* using a stimulant to jumpstart your metabolism. Fen-Phen consisted of two medications working together to augment each other's effectiveness. The combination was supposed to be the magic bullet that would result in a good amount of weight loss for patients with relative ease. It seemed too good to be true. Lots of people used Fen-Phen in the hope that it would provide a solution for weight loss. However, it didn't take long before serious heart complications began to surface among those using the medication, and Fen-Phen's promises evaporated right before our eyes. This saga left us with a typical cautionary tale of how taking something difficult like losing weight and making it as easy as taking a pill is usually not good. Two decades later, Fen-Phen is still regularly talked about as a horror story of medical weight loss.

But the Fen-Phen story isn't over yet! The complications of Fen-Phen were primarily blamed on one of the two medications, fenfluramine, which was thought to be the root cause of the heart issues. The second component, phentermine (Phen), was thought to be safe. So, once the stigma wore off a bit, phentermine became commercially available as a prescription medication for weight loss. Patients should have an EKG before starting the medication and be monitored throughout the course of treatment. This medication acts like a stimulant and causes the typical side effects that we see with all stimulants. However, the societal pressure to control weight is so strong that patients still ask for this medication by name (Adipex-P or phentermine). In the last decade, I've used this medication many times with patients with varying degrees of success. Based on their published data though, the best-case scenario is that a patient can expect to lose three to seven percent of their total body weight. That's not insignificant, but it also isn't life-changing—and probably not worth the risk of long-term damage to your health.

Another cautionary tale comes from Alli (orlistat), which was approved by the FDA for weight loss in 2007. This medication works in a completely different fashion than Fen-Phen or phentermine to help with weight loss. It reduces the body's ability to absorb fat, which once again seems to make a lot of sense. Practically, though, Alli doesn't work out nicely and proved to be less effective than promised. Because the lower GI tract can't handle undigested fat, a bad case of diarrhea develops every time the GI tract comes in contact with undigested fat. The situation was so urgent (think uncontrollable) that the package insert recommended bringing a change of clothes with you when using the medication. That is gross. Many of us want to lose weight, but very few of us are willing to tolerate accidents and embarrassment like that. The FDA also listed "oily spotting" as a known side effect; you can imagine for yourself what that entails. As a result of these horrific side effects, the medication never really became popular or had widespread use. It is still available under a different name today.

Both examples illustrate that there is a huge demand (or need) for weight loss medication. It also highlights that the general public is willing to tolerate a wide range of side effects to accomplish losing weight. This speaks volumes to the societal pressures that make individuals want to lose weight but are not able to make the lifestyle modifications needed to accomplish significant lasting weight loss.

Our weight defines a lot about our lives and how others perceive us. Sometimes, individuals who don't struggle with weight issues make hurtful comments to individuals who do. The thought of excessive hunger and constant overeating just doesn't make sense to some because they have been blessed with weak receptors for the hunger hormones. They genuinely do not feel the same hunger intensity some individuals experience. Therefore, they have more control over their eating habits because hunger doesn't affect them as strongly. It does appear that obesity is a disorder of physiology in some individuals; it's not just that certain people overeat due to lack of self-control or willpower.

Appetite suppressants have been available for almost thirty years now. They don't seem to work though, because we often eat not because we are hungry, but because we are happy, sad, anxious, smell food, see food, or think about food. This is emotional eating. Therefore, it's not just our appetite that drives us to be overweight even though that is a significant part of it. Something else is going on in some people's bodies that drives them to eat more and gain weight at an above average rate.

That leads us to explore what a perfect weight loss medication would look like. What would make someone lose weight in a relatively easy fashion while not causing horrible side effects? Certainly, exercise and a healthy diet would be part of the medical regimen, but what would we look for in the perfect weight loss medication? We would need not only an appetite suppressant but also a way to make it easy to stop putting food in our mouths due to an emotional response. To stop emotional eating, the ideal medication would not only need to suppress the appetite so we aren't hungry all the time, but it also would need to create a feeling of being full or satisfied. While we are dreaming . . . the ideal medication would need to "trick" our bodies into burning fat when we take it (like intermittent fasting or ketosis does) to provide a quicker result as well. A medication having all these qualities seems too good to be true! Consequently, we are back to needing lifestyle changes to accomplish long-term weight loss, and those changes are notoriously hard to accomplish and stick to.

In the past, I was not willing to cross that bridge and try weight loss medications. Their side effects and potential long-term health damage were driven into me during medical school. The risk just wasn't worth it. During medical school and residency, I was taught that just taking in fewer calories than you burn every day would result in weight loss. I was told that it really wasn't more complicated than that. People who are overweight just don't have the willpower to say no to food and lose weight, according to the general understanding of weight. Even as I struggled to control my own weight, I stuck to those principles that were ingrained in me during my medical training.

I would write prescriptions for weight loss medications for patients and watch them continue to struggle. Successes were few and far in between the many failures. I often felt like patients were just throwing their money away for the hope of weight loss; the tools (medications) available were just not able to help them in any meaningful way. We would have them do all the right things, meet with a dietitian, and track their exercise. But like most people, they could only fight this battle for so long before they eventually gave in and went back to old habits. I was left with a helpless feeling for these patients.

Personally though, I felt the effects of this constant battle that we all were losing. Another notch in the belt to let out, going up another size in my pants, constantly having my shirts fit too tight. Slowly, I came to accept that this was life; it was what was supposed to happen. After all, most people gain four pounds a year, so why would I be any different? I was on track to becoming obese and had mentally accepted that. It's so strange how we can justify anything to ourselves even when we know better than to believe what we are telling ourselves. I came to accept that moving forward, my life would involve weight-related health issues. Getting a joint replacement wouldn't be so bad, right? Most Americans end up with a stent in their coronary arteries, right? I could always find someone who weighed more than me, so I could rationalize that I wasn't as bad as they were. This all made me feel comfortable accepting the fact that I was giving up the battle. Slowly but surely, I was justifying to myself that it was OK for me to become obese.

Accepting this hopeless feeling had devastating consequences. I resigned myself to being someone who was overweight and would eventually become obese. That opened the door for me to overeat more and more. After all, if I was doomed to be obese, I might as well enjoy the food along the way and eat a little more. It wasn't healthy, but I had fought the battle for so long with no long-lasting success. Every win was quickly followed by even more weight gain. It was an impossible battle, and I just wanted it to be done. Plus, overeating caused that dopamine release in the brain, which made me feel good. So overeating was becoming more of a "joy" in my life. It was easier for me to resign myself to becoming obese and dealing with all the health consequences that came along with that. I was unable to exercise myself to a normal weight; I was unable to calorie-restrict myself into a normal weight; and I began to not care about it anymore. Not only was my physical health suffering, but my mental health was suffering as well. Moreover, my children were watching and thinking that this was normal behavior—that gaining weight was inevitable. Making hard, healthier decisions with food just wasn't worth it, and it was better to give in and enjoy what you could. I was shaping their view of healthy choices without even realizing it . . . or caring about it.

I could not fathom a future that didn't involve me being overweight. There was no reality where I lost the extra weight and kept it off. To be able to do that was so far out of the realm of reality that it was incomprehensible to me. That was my future . . . not only had I become OK with being overweight and slowly becoming obese, but I had also accepted it and began to embrace it. I saw knee replacements in my future; I saw multiple pharmaceutical medications that would hopefully control my chronic conditions of high blood pressure and high cholesterol. I could treat those things for patients, and it wouldn't be so bad for me to have them treated. I wouldn't need to ever be rated as extra healthy for life insurance, so what did it matter after all? With modern medicine, I would still live long enough to see my kids grow up and have kids. Life would still be good for me; I would just be overweight and eventually obese. That was the picture of my life that I had accepted moving forward, and I would be happy with it. There just wasn't another path forward that I could find to change this. Talking to patients, I realized I wasn't alone in these feelings, but it would take a miracle to change things. It would take something that didn't exist, something miraculous—something too good to be true, a game changer to change my trajectory.

KEY POINTS

☞ Everyone wants a simple weight loss pill.

> ➤ Society has tried several without much success.

> ➤ Appetite suppression is good in theory but doesn't seem to work in pill form.

☞ Emotions and hormones interfere with our relationship with food.

☞ It's easier to accept the status quo of weight gain.

> ➤ Change requires work.

Chapter 3

A NEW BREAKTHROUGH – IS IT TOO GOOD TO BE TRUE?

In 2005, Byetta (exenatide) got Federal Drug Administration (FDA) approval. This was the first medication in a new class of medications called Glucagon-Like Peptide-1, or GLP-1 for short, used for the treatment of diabetes. In addition to helping the body process insulin and regulate blood sugar, this medication slowed down digestion and promoted a feeling of fullness. As these medications were used to treat diabetes, an interesting side effect became apparent as the patients began losing weight.

These medications stem from the discovery of the natural GLP-1 hormone in the early 1980s. When the body secretes this hormone, it causes more insulin to be made, which in turn lowers blood sugar. But interestingly, manipulating this hormone didn't cause the horrible side effect of extremely low blood sugar (hypoglycemia) as most other diabetic medications do. It only caused insulin production in proportion to the glucose level, thereby avoiding the side effect of low blood sugar. This means that one of the common and most disabling side effects of treating diabetes (i.e., loss of consciousness) could be avoided. Moreover, this hormone makes the liver slow down its sugar production, which improves "fatty liver disease," which is becoming more common in American adults.

Five years later, in 2010, the FDA approved a second GLP-1 medication Victoza (liraglutide) to be used to treat diabetes. The race was on and soon, there would be many different flavors of these medications. The treatment of diabetes was revolutionized by this class of medications. Researchers developed extended-release formulas and also tried oral forms of the medicines versus the original injectable. However, oral forms proved to be less effective in general.

The hype of this class of medications only increased when it was discovered that they could also be used to reduce the risk of cardiovascular disease. That's right, taking a diabetic medication could lower your risk of heart attacks and strokes. Think about the potential of that discovery. Cardiovascular disease (heart attacks and strokes) is so prevalent in our society that the opportunity to lower the occurrence would have a tremendous impact on our future.

Victoza became a pioneer by using this class of medications in non-diabetic patients. Could these medications produce weight loss along with other benefits in patients who don't have diabetes? Certainly, weight loss and a reduced cardiovascular disease risk would be appealing to non-diabetic patients. Plus, not having the risk of causing low blood sugar levels made it an interesting question. Victoza (liraglutide) answered that question in 2014 when they got FDA approval for weight management in obese individuals or overweight individuals with a weight-related medical condition. Victoza was rebranded as Saxenda, and a new era in weight management was launched.

Saxenda wasn't perfect by any means. It required a daily injection and had to be kept refrigerated. The weight loss wasn't great, but it was the best we had experienced from a medication to that point. In 2017 though, Ozempic (Semaglutide), which is similar to Victoza but requires only a weekly injection, was introduced for the treatment of diabetes. In 2021, it was rebranded and brought to market as Wegovy after getting FDA approval for weight loss. It showed significantly more weight loss potential and had an even more favorable side effect profile.

Then in 2022, Mounjaro (tirzepatide) was approved for the treatment of diabetes, and the trials showed a weight reduction of sixteen to twenty-two percent. That's life-changing—a game changer for obesity and weight management. Some patients lost over 100 pounds in the clinical trials. As an added benefit that encouraged individuals to continue on their weight loss journey, most of the weight loss comes in the first few months of using the medication. In November 2023, tirzepatide was approved by the FDA for weight loss under the new brand name Zepbound.

Side Effects

Although these medications appear to be very promising, it isn't all rainbows and sunshine. The medications can have potent side effects. They slow down GI tract transit, so they can cause nausea and vomiting, abdominal pain, and constipation (or diarrhea if taken orally). Though rare, they can inflame the pancreas and lead to pancreatitis. And there is a 900-pound gorilla in the room about whether they might cause a very specific type of thyroid cancer. Yikes!

All medications have a side effect profile; therefore, the risk and benefits must be weighed before starting any medication. These medications are no different. But is the risk of thyroid cancer worth taking the medication to lose weight? Well, it's not just some weight . . . it can be up to twenty percent of your total body weight. That's a big game changer, and we know the long-term health **benefits** from that kind of weight loss.

Risk versus Benefits

Let's dive into the thyroid cancer risk more because that is what patients seem to gravitate to after doing their own research on these medications. Almost all the other side effects are mild, and when patients complain to me about them, my first response is, "Let's just stop the medication," but patients don't want to do that. They are seeing the results of the weight loss and want to work out a solution to deal with the side effects or manage them rather than just stop the medication and have the weight loss end.

Cancer is scary and as a society, we have taken great lengths to lessen the population's risk of certain kinds of cancers. So, are we willing to inject ourselves with a medication that might cause cancer if it means we end up skinnier?

In the Victoza (liraglutide) clinical trials using mice, the mice who were given the medication had a higher risk of developing a specific kind of thyroid cancer when compared to the ones who did not get the medication. The human trials though, did not demonstrate this link although there were still some concerns. As a result, the FDA concluded that there is not enough evidence to determine one way or the other. But if there is a potential risk, it is a very small risk. Moreover, routine thyroid cancer screening was not even recommended for individuals using these medications.

The other GLP-1 medications did not show this risk. And the best evidence currently does not show a causal relationship between GLP-1 medications and thyroid cancers. However, because they all belong to the same class of medications, they all carry the same risk warning from the FDA. Even though some individuals taking GLP-1 medications have contracted thyroid cancer, the incidence of cases does not outpace the incidence in the general population. Therefore, it could be that the mice in the original Victoza studies were more prone to thyroid cancer for a genetic reason, rather than Victoza causing thyroid cancer. It is difficult to know for sure, but that's my opinion after examining the evidence.

Doctors weigh such risks against the benefits of every medication before writing a prescription. These GLP-1 medications provide the benefit of weight loss, and the weight loss itself has additional well-known benefits. Being at an appropriate weight lowers your risk of illnesses such as heart attacks, strokes, high blood pressure, high cholesterol, diabetes, and arthritis. We also know that carrying around extra weight significantly hurts our long-term health. In my practice, I see my patients every year for an annual physical during which I spend time talking about the benefits of weight loss. So, the fact that these medications cause weight loss should be factored into the decision about whether to use these medications ourselves or for our patients.

Early Results with GLP-1 Medicines

The difficulty with practicing medicine is that medications don't all work the same in every individual. When I start a patient on a blood pressure medicine, I always have them come back into the office and recheck their blood pressure after a few weeks on the medicine because I can't be sure that it is going to work or how well it will work. That's the art of practicing medicine . . . constantly adjusting to how the patient is responding to both the disease process and the medication. Therefore, when I started using GLP-1 medications for weight loss with patients, I expected the same thing. I expected some patients to have great success, others to have a small amount of weight loss, and some to not have any weight loss. But that's not what I saw; instead, most patients lost weight. It wasn't a question of "if" patients would lose weight on these medications; it was a question of "how much" weight a patient would lose on these medications. It started to seem too good to be true . . . and we all know the saying that if something is too good to be true, then it's probably not true.

But I also observed something else that was surprising. Patients were happy; their mental health was improving. I'm not talking about patients with serious psychiatric disorders. I'm referencing patients who had admitted to themselves (like I had) that they were always going to be overweight or obese and that life was always going to be like this for them. After a few months on a GLP-1 medication as they started to lose weight, they began to view their future differently. Perhaps they weren't always going to be obese individuals. They had hope on their horizon again . . . and we all could use more hope in our lives. They were excited about their future, which they hadn't been excited about for years. I'm a firm believer that when an individual starts losing sight of hope for their future, that's when bad things start to happen.

Something else changed as more of my patients began using these medications. My own job satisfaction improved. As a physician, I often encounter patients who are either having a bad day or the worst day of their lives. When patients reach out to their doctor, most of the time it's not because they are feeling wonderful and just wanted to let the doctor know how great they feel. No. Patients reach out in a time of crisis or when they are very symptomatic with an illness. But patients on GLP-1 medications were reaching out to me just to check in and let me know that they had lost five, ten, or fifteen pounds. They would reach out and let me know that they reached their first weight loss goal and were excited about trying to reach their next goal. This happened over and over again with multiple patients . . . and it began affecting me. My job satisfaction was improving, and I selfishly liked it. These were patients I had helped in the worst days of their lives as they dealt with major illnesses and struggles, and it made me so happy to see them succeeding. But it made me happier to know that they were improving their long-term health too. They didn't even comprehend how much better their health was going to be for years to come because they were able to lose so much weight. They were going to have a much better retirement because of this huge accomplishment. Most patients were focused on short-term improvements. But they found even more joy when I reviewed their updated labs with them and took the time to explain with objective data how much better their long-term health was going to be because they were able to lose weight.

My Weight Loss Journey

I set a goal to lose thirty pounds over twelve months. I started exercising more regularly and reducing calories in my diet.

I looked for ways to be more active in my day-to-day life. I started riding a bike for my ten-mile commute to work instead of driving, and I started using a standing desk while at work. I was slowly losing weight with these changes, but it was also costing me something that my wife and kids would point out. I was "hangry" from being hungry all the time. I was sleeping less because I was waking up early to exercise, so I was tired all the time and wasn't fun to be around anymore. Trying to lose weight was negatively impacting the people I valued most—my wife and kids. After three months of doing this, I began to wonder if I should try a GLP-1 medication. I was able to lose seven pounds on my own after three months, so I was on track to reach my goal of losing thirty pounds in a year. But could I lose weight without harming the relationships with the people I valued most? I had a front row seat to multiple patients losing weight from these medications. And so, I wondered whether it was time for me to find out if they really were too good to be true.

Before we explore that option though, we need to take a closer look at the cardiovascular risk reduction. This is a groundbreaking change in how we view weight loss medications and what they can offer. I also believe it holds the key to having these medications receive widespread adoption and usage (along with insurance approval). Before we go further, we need to slow down and examine cardiovascular risk.

KEY POINTS

- ☞ GLP-1 medications have a huge potential to fix the obesity epidemic.
- ☞ Multiple generations of these medications are available.
- ☞ They all have side effects and risks.
  - › Not losing weight has risks as well.
- ☞ GLP-1 medications have huge potential physical and emotional benefits.

Chapter 4

CHANGES IN CARDIOVASCULAR DISEASE RISKS

The benefits of these GLP-1 medications go beyond just losing weight, vanity, and helping your joints last longer. They also significantly improve your overall health, both in the short term and long term. One major benefit is the reduction in the risk of cardiovascular disease for patients on these medications. Cardiovascular disease usually leads to a heart attack, known in the medical community as a myocardial infarction. A heart attack occurs when the body lays down plaque in the coronary arteries that builds up or breaks off, completely occluding blood flow downstream. Without adequate blood flow, the downstream tissue (heart muscle in the coronary arteries) becomes ischemic and ultimately dies without aggressive treatment. This process not only happens in the heart but it can also happen in the brain when plaque breaks off and goes downstream to the arteries that supply the brain. When this plaque occludes blood flow in the brain, it is called a stroke, or cerebral vascular accident (CVA in the medical community). But cardiovascular disease doesn't just affect the heart and brain, our entire bodies are fed by the cardiovascular system through a series of arteries. Lots of those arteries can develop plaque that ruptures and occludes blood flow downstream; this problem can happen in the legs or anywhere in the body. Cardiovascular disease is the leading killer in America, so any reduction in that risk can make a huge impact for our bodies and society as a whole.

You might think that you exercise and eat healthy, so cardiovascular disease isn't a risk for you, but you would be wrong. Yes, diet and exercise are part of the equation, but genetics makes up a big part of the equation too. And you can't do anything to change your genetics. Almost every American is at risk for cardiovascular disease despite their lifestyle. A heart-healthy lifestyle with generous amounts of exercise and a pristine diet might delay the onset of plaque, but it won't negate it all together. The proof of that comes in the realization that this process can start in childhood as early as age two. You read that right, the medical community has discovered that plaque is being laid down in the arteries of some children as young as two years old. We are all at risk from this process, and it must be taken seriously when deciding how aggressively to undertake a weight loss program with or without medication.

Statins (e.g., simvastatin, atorvastatin, rosuvastatin) were previously one of the best medications we had to treat cardiovascular disease. Not only did they lower cholesterol levels, but they also helped stabilize plaque (i.e., turn soft plaque into hard plaque), which lowers cardiovascular disease risks. Hard plaque is less likely to break off and cause downstream occlusions than soft plaque. With long-term, constant use, statins have also been shown to cause plaque regression. With the help of a statin, it is possible to lower the plaque burden in your arteries. That takes a long time, and you have to be dedicated to taking the medication and living a heart-healthy lifestyle. For many years, statins were the gold standard for lowering your cardiovascular disease risk.

Recently, a newer class of medications called PCSK9 inhibitors became available. These injectable medications (e.g., Repatha and Praluent) can drive down LDL (bad) cholesterol levels into the single digits. They are generally well-tolerated but are extraordinarily expensive, and getting them approved through insurance can be difficult. Therefore, PCSK9 inhibitors are used more as a last resort medication rather than a first- or second-line option. Even though they work tremendously well, insurance companies have put up a big hurdle to using them in clinical practice. It is possible to get them approved for treating cardiovascular disease but trying to get insurance approval to use them for prevention is a fool's errand.

Talking about all these medications illustrates the point that there are many good options for treating cardiovascular disease after coronary arteries have been damaged. But imagine how much better it is to be proactive with your cardiovascular health. What would it be like if you could prevent cardiovascular disease from occurring in the first place? Weight loss, especially weight loss with GLP-1 medications like Ozempic and Mounjaro can help get things under control and hopefully prevent cardiovascular disease from occurring if they are taken early enough. I don't think they will be the magic cure-all, but they represent a paradigm shift of focusing on prevention and early treatment, rather than waiting for a problem to occur and then trying to fix it. Preventing the number one killer in America certainly is enough to get anyone excited, right?

For most people, that is enough to tip the scales of whether you should use GLP-1s even if they are not morbidly obese. The most common concern I get when discussing these medications with patients is that we don't know their long-term risk. And I agree with that completely. However, there is a risk of doing nothing. But even more, we already know the risks of carrying around an extra twenty or thirty pounds. So, the risk-benefit ratio has to incorporate the risks of keeping that extra weight . . . not just on your heart, but on every system in your body, including your joints. Losing twenty to thirty pounds will significantly improve your blood pressure, lower your cholesterol, stabilize your blood sugar levels, help your insulin metabolism, and even avoid becoming prediabetic—whether you lose weight with medication or without medication. But most Americans have already had their entire adult life up to this point to lose that weight and haven't been successful. If these medications can help you be successful with weight loss and reduce the risk that any of those devastating things will happen to you, that must be part of the equation. I agree that this risk reduction seems almost too good to be true. It does seem incredible that one medication can address multiple problems *and* work on the root cause, which is excess weight. It is a game changer!

Even more eye-opening is the fact that mice who are calorie restricted live longer than mice who get to eat more calories. This has been a long-known conundrum in the medical community. Most mammals thrive and live longer when they are severely calorie restricted. There haven't been human trials on this for obvious reasons, so we need to assume that humans respond the same way as all the other mammals. But to me, that's not an unreasonable assumption. There seems to be some sort of positive stress on the body that enables it to function better when calories are in limited supply. We saw this on a minor scale with intermittent fasting. Fasting for sixteen to eighteen hours a day brought about many health benefits beyond just weight loss. Now think of the average American diet and lifestyle. Excess calories are abundant and all around us. That makes not overconsuming exceedingly difficult. We like to celebrate with food, mourn with food, laugh with food, and bond with food—all while we don't need those extra calories. They are just comfort (remember dopamine release in our brains?) for us in different situations.

One of the ways that GLP-1 medications are thought to decrease cardiovascular disease risk is through the utilization and reduction of visceral fat. Visceral fat is the fat on the inside of your body that surrounds your organs. It is a layer of warmth, but it is also a way to store unused calories. GLP-1 medications seem to cause a higher rate of visceral fat loss than would be expected with typical weight loss. And just like with total body weight loss, we already know the long-term benefits of having a lower amount of visceral fat: fewer heart attacks, fewer strokes, and lower risks of some gastrointestinal cancers.

The benefits of lowering the risk of cardiovascular disease, regardless of which method is used (natural or pharmaceutical) are well-documented and well-known. GLP-1 medications are becoming important tools that we can use to lower that long-term risk. Hopefully, we will see that play out with significantly fewer heart attacks and strokes in the coming years as these medications are more widely adopted and utilized. We should also see less of the other weight-related comorbidities. Can you imagine how many fewer joint replacements we would need if fewer overweight people were stressing their joints with every step they take?

And there are so many more benefits to these medications besides just weight reduction and lower cardiovascular disease risk. Both tangible and intangible benefits arise in patients who successfully use these medications to augment their weight loss program. Yes, they will see better health, but they also notice improvements in areas of their life they weren't expecting. With twenty to thirty pounds gone, they have more energy to do things that they didn't think they could do anymore, such as playing with children or grandchildren, being active outdoors, traveling, having a new outlook on life, and more. Patients have also reported that they seem to have a clearer or sharper thought process too. They can work things out in their minds better after losing weight and can recall things quicker.

By far, though, my favorite part of talking to these patients is exploring the mental health benefits with them. They are happier, and they feel accomplished because they have finally completed a goal they have struggled with for years. After that accomplishment, they often keep the momentum going and tackle other areas of their lives that need improvement. This one win with their weight leads to another win in a different aspect of their life, which leads to yet another win somewhere else. That confidence bleeds over into every aspect of their physical and mental health. It's a great cycle to see in their lives, and it helps them maintain their weight loss after they stop the medications. What we are really interested in is making those lifestyle modifications that make these changes sustainable for the rest of your life.

KEY POINTS

- ☛ Cardiovascular disease is prevalent and can affect anyone.

- ☛ There are several different ways to manage cardiovascular disease with medications.

- ☛ Weight loss lowers the risk of cardiovascular disease.

- ☛ This is true for weight loss from medications too.

  › Calorie restriction has benefits on lifespan.

- ☛ Mental and emotional health is tied to weight loss and overall health.

Chapter 5

FAST VERSUS SLOW WEIGHT LOSS . . . WHICH IS BETTER?

I remember the day I decided to ask one of my partners to consider writing me a prescription for Mounjaro, which is a GLP-1 medication. We have a body composition scale at our office, so it didn't take a lot of convincing because there was no excuse about my weight all being muscle or my being big-boned (whatever that means). The objective data was clear: I was severely overweight and headed toward obesity. I had high blood pressure and high cholesterol—two weight-related conditions. I had tried numerous times to lose weight with minimal success, which never lasted. It was obvious the trendline for my weight and waist was upward. There wasn't a way in sight for me to fix the problem on my own without compromising the relationships I valued most.

After I got the medication from the pharmacy, I was somewhat embarrassed about it. I didn't tell my wife before

I did my first injection because of this uncomfortable feeling. I'm not quite sure why I felt that way, but I did. I think it was rooted in two things, first admitting that I had let myself get to the point that I needed a pharmaceutical medication to lose weight and second that I was giving up on my own ability to accomplish weight loss on my own. After a decade of telling patients day in and day out that diet and exercise were the only ways to lose weight, I was now searching for a different way. I had come to the point where I needed help, and I was ready to get the help—in the form of an expensive injection.

I love ice cream and I don't think I had ever said no to ice cream in my life. I regularly ate a big bowl of ice cream several nights a week, and I didn't care if ice cream shortened my life because it tasted so good. I would also look for reasons to have ice cream, and my kids knew that if they asked Daddy for ice cream, I would say that we all could (should) have it. It was an emotional comfort to me, and I didn't even realize it. It took me back to my childhood, and I loved it. My wife would even say that I was addicted to ice cream in the same way I was addicted to drinking soda.

The first day I gave myself an injection we already had plans to walk to a favorite local ice cream shop as a family that evening. I remember vividly feeling that there was absolutely no way I could put ice cream (or anything else) in my mouth. I felt so stuffed that I could not get ice cream that night. Never before in my life had I ever turned down ice cream, but that night, things changed for me. My wife and kids knew something was up if I wasn't going to get ice cream and that was the end of keeping the fact that I was using the medication a secret.

I lost twenty pounds in the first month on the medication. This was too good to be true! I went from my clothes being too tight to having loose clothes that were literally falling off me. I liked the way I felt in my clothes for the first time in many years. The speed of the weight loss was unbelievable. I was experiencing firsthand what many of my patients had already told me about. This was all too good to be true!

I also noticed that I had my willpower back; I no longer felt addicted to food like I used to be. Previously, I had used food as a reward; after a hard day, I would reward myself with a treat. While on the medication, that reward feeling wasn't there anymore. I was able to make healthy changes to what and how much I was eating. I was able to give up drinking soda almost overnight whereas, I had struggled numerous times before to stop drinking soda. I was seeing many significant benefits to being on tirzepatide (Mounjaro/Zepbound).

In three months, I lost fifty pounds on the medication and needed to stop it because I was running out of weight to lose. I blew past my original goal of losing thirty pounds. Never did I imagine losing fifty pounds. But there is not much data on how to wean off these medications or how to set up a maintenance regimen. I had a new problem. What should I do next? Certainly, stopping the medication would result in weight gain. There is data to suggest that you will gain six to eight percent of your total body weight back after you go off the medication. I was nervous about cutting it out completely or starting a pattern of ups and downs with my weight.

Developing a Better Relationship with Food

Traditionally, doctors have taught that it is better to lose weight slowly. That is, the more slowly you lose weight, the more likely you are to keep it off. Knowing that I had lost so much weight in a short time made me feel like I was set up for a big disappointment and that I would regain most (or maybe even more) of the weight back. GLP-1 medications are unique in that they cause a large amount of weight loss in a short amount of time. Generally, in the first two to three months, patients lose most of their weight. Are we just setting patients up to yo-yo and worse yet, give them false hope and false reassurance?

I took the approach of spacing out the injections to retrain myself on how to have a healthy relationship with food and to learn how much food to eat (which is vastly different from what our society tells us). I viewed the medication as my training wheels and as an opportunity to shrink my stomach. The stomach is a muscle, and it can get stretched out and expand, but it can also contract and shrink. If the medication would make it easier for me to shrink my stomach, perhaps I could continue to keep the weight off after the medication without all the struggles from before.

Using those two ideas, the medication was training wheels for me to relearn how to have a better relationship with food and help shrink my stomach. I used the medication for a short time and tried to maintain the weight loss on my own without using medication. It seemed to make a difference, and I was able to keep the weight off. Perhaps our old thought process of slow weight loss was not valid anymore with the advent of these new medications. These two ideas had forced me to make lifestyle changes that I always talk to patients about. The medication had made it *easy* to make these lifestyle changes and increased the likelihood that I will be able to sustain these valuable key changes indefinitely. It certainly seemed to be a real game changer!

But this brings up a valuable point; these medications are relatively new, and we don't have lots of data about how to stop the medication, wean off the medication, or make a maintenance regimen with the medication. There are still a lot of unknowns. I had invested a significant amount of money and accepted the possibility of unknown risks to experiment with these medications. I wanted the weight loss to persist as long as possible—for the rest of my life. Without decades of data though, how would this be possible?

I really liked the idea of spacing out the injections because that allowed me to try life without the medication but in a "safe" environment. This strategy gave me the grace to experiment with short breaks from the medication while knowing that I would resume the medication soon. This worked very well for me. I was able to stop the medication completely with this mindset. However, I do have patients who prefer to stay on a once-a-month dosing regimen (instead of weekly) to help maintain their weight loss. I don't see anything wrong with that idea as long as they are staying healthy doing it. Having access to a body composition scale helps with monitoring to be sure they aren't unknowingly hurting themselves.

Keeping the Weight Off

The other big hurdle to overcome has to do with the set point theory for weight loss. You may be familiar with people who lose weight and then seemingly keep doing everything right only to gain the weight back. This was part of the reason why the medical community believed that slow weight loss is better. The set point theory for weight proposes that each of our bodies has a weight that it wants to maintain. You can work really hard and lose a few pounds, but your body is going to go back to its preferred set point. It is very difficult to change that set point. That also explains why you can overeat for a couple days and only gain a few pounds that end up going away after a few days. So, a calorie is not always equivalent to any other calorie.

As a result of the set point theory, the medical community started pushing patients to lose weight slowly. It takes time to change your set point, so you need to slowly lose weight to change it. But GLP-1 medications cause the greatest weight loss in the first few months. Our best guess is that you need to sustain weight loss for a year before you can permanently change your set point for weight. Losing weight slowly will encourage your body to have a lower set point to return to if you gain the weight back, which most of us who lose weight do. Thus, slower weight loss would result in you keeping some of the weight off and "rebounding" to a lower weight than previously when the weight comes back. So how do I reconcile the reality of GLP-1 medications with our view of weight loss and the set point theory?

That's when I went back to the basic biology I learned in medical school. The stomach is a muscle, which can be expanded, but it also can be shrunk. In our society and culture, we tend to overeat. Portion sizes are out of control. As a result, we have unknowingly stretched out our stomachs, so it takes more food to make us feel full. With the thought that a smaller stomach would help me sustain weight loss, I utilized the ease of losing weight by controlling hunger and making me feel full to shrink my stomach. This "smaller" stomach would last after I stopped the medication completely and hopefully, it would help me maintain the lower weight, despite losing the weight so quickly. Prior to introducing GLP-1 medications to my patients, I routinely talked to them about this to aid them in their weight loss attempts. I encourage them to strive to shrink their stomach as they lose weight. But the reality is that to shrink your stomach to a more appropriate size, you must be hungry for long periods of time. So, it was never a fun conversation to have with patients. No one wants to do the hard work of weight loss **and** constantly feel hungry too. Therefore, very few people were able to apply this concept prior to using the medications.

GLP-1 medications not only suppress your appetite, but they also promote the feeling of fullness. They are great medications to utilize as you attempt to shrink your stomach to a more appropriate size because you won't constantly feel hungry while doing so. I utilized this strategy and had great success. Not only did the medication help me lose weight, but the effects of the medication helped me keep the weight off after I stopped the medication. In turn, I should be able to keep the weight off for a much longer time and have my set point continually get lower as I sustain the weight loss. So as old habits creep back in and the societal pressures become harder to resist, I would migrate back to a lower weight than I started with. This was all a theory that came from utilizing the medical knowledge, education, and experience I had accumulated over the years. I hoped that I wouldn't be throwing time, money, and energy away with this weight loss plan.

KEY POINTS

☛ Slow weight loss was the standard for years.

☛ Along with fast weight loss comes the need to learn and apply the set point theory.

☛ The medications work best when you think of them as training wheels:

> ➤ Relearn your relationship with food.

> ➤ Making lifestyle changes is easier with the medications.

Chapter 6

WEIGHT LOSS IS NOT ALL RAINBOWS AND SUNSHINE

Even though I utilized my knowledge and the new medications to lose weight, it was still challenging. I had to struggle through the unnatural process of weight loss, break through plateaus, and fight addictions. This was work although it was easier work than when I tried to lose weight in the past.

Coping with the Unnatural Process of Weight Loss

The problem with weight loss is that our bodies are designed to retain every calorie we put in our mouths. It's only been in the last 100 years or so that food has become abundant for civilization. For the vast history of mankind, humans lived without an abundance of food; they had to work hard to forage for their food. People had meals sporadically and as a result, their bodies became extremely efficientat absorbing and retaining calories (as fat). Then when food started to become easily available and abundant, we started to gain weight as a natural result of the years of adaptation to living with a scarcity of food. This, coupled with our lifestyles becoming more sedentary and our food becoming more calorie-dense led to the obesity epidemic we are witnessing around us.

Those are not the only reasons we are struggling with an obesity epidemic though. Weight loss is unnatural for our bodies; therefore, we are trying to force our bodies to do something that they were never designed to do. This resistance, coupled with the set point theory discussed in the last chapter, is why we encounter plateaus when we try to lose weight. A plateau happens when you are doing everything right—taking in fewer calories, exercising, and sleeping well—but you aren't losing pounds on the scale. Even with these new GLP-1 medications for weight loss, you will still encounter plateaus, which can be very frustrating.

Breaking Through Plateaus

Weight loss curves that show a gradual loss of weight are very misleading. Instead, a weight loss graph should look more like stair steps. You are stuck on a step for a while and then you have a free fall of sorts to the next step. At each step, your body is doing everything it can to hold onto the extra calories stored as fat. The body is a beautiful creation, so it gets better and better over time at holding onto these extra calories. Your body literally adapts to the new level and works against the weight loss you are trying to accomplish because for most of human history, food was scarce. Therefore, each plateau or step takes longer (or is harder) to break through. The medication might make it easier to keep doing the right thing, but there is no way to shortcut this process. Any weight loss journey will involve frustrating plateaus that last longer and become harder to break through each time.

Plateaus can get into your thought process and make you feel like you are doing something wrong. They can certainly make you want to give up on the weight loss journey. Without medication, this is when I see patients give up and resort to their previous habits without making any permanent lifestyle changes. But knowing that you will encounter plateaus and that they will last longer each time you encounter them can help you stay focused and on track. Plateaus are an evolutionary good thing. They helped our ancestors survive when food was not readily available—when most people did not know when or where their next meal would come from.

Rethinking Protein Intake

One of the key pieces of advice I discuss with my patients is to rethink the kinds of food in their diets. Most of us were taught some version of the food pyramid growing up. Grains or carbohydrates were on the bottom, and proteins were on the top of the pyramid. We were taught to eat more grains and that we don't need all that much protein each day. The problem with that thinking is that it doesn't fit in today's world. When the food pyramid was pushed on our society, the forces at play were drastically different than they are now, and protein is more readily available for us than ever before. Grains and carbs are a cheap and easy way to get calories and the full feeling. But they aren't the best thing to consume, especially if you are trying to lose weight. I'll stay away from the gluten sensitivity or pro-inflammatory argument of carbs for now. But no matter how you look at it, most of us consume too many carbohydrates.

So, if the food pyramid isn't a good thing to follow, what should you be consuming on a day-to-day basis? The answer to that question is protein—and more protein than you think. The current recommendations vary widely for just how much protein you should be taking in; some authorities go up to one gram of protein per kilogram of body weight (that's about 70 grams of protein for the average adult). You may find it difficult to consume that much protein each day unless you change a lot of things in your diet. As you make those changes in your diet, you quickly realize that consuming more protein has the side effect of making you feel full quicker, and it gives a more lasting full feeling. Therefore, if you utilize the GLP-1 medications with this idea, you will feel full longer from the medication and the calories you consume. This will enable you to seize the opportunity to shrink your stomach. Even while on the medication, filling your stomach with protein instead of carbohydrates will create less actual volume in your stomach. Your stomach will start to shrink and hopefully provide another helpful key to keeping the weight off after you stop the medication. This is a key lifestyle change that will help you get long-lasting results.

Protecting Muscle Mass

I'm not saying that a person should **only** eat protein, but you should start paying attention to the amount of protein you consume daily. Most people need to increase their amount of protein to keep up with these new guidelines. This also serves an additional purpose. If you aren't careful with the GLP-1 class of medications, you can lose muscle instead of body fat. That would put you in a worse metabolic state than when you began even though you have lost pounds. This topic illustrates another important idea about our bodies and weight loss: protein is vitally important to your body, and if you don't consume it, your body will break down your own muscles to get the protein it needs. A person who loses twenty pounds hasn't done themselves any favor if ten of those pounds are muscle mass. In fact, they may be in a worse metabolic situation than before losing twenty pounds. Protein is vital for survival, and our bodies will consume it one way or another . . . even from our own muscles if we don't take in enough from our diets.

A high protein diet is different from the popular Carnivore diet or Atkins diet. Don't solely consume protein; eat fruits and vegetables as well. Always start with protein for a meal and add in the fruits or vegetables. I know some fruits and vegetables have carbohydrates, and we just discussed the lack of nutritional value in carbohydrates. I firmly believe that the carbohydrates in fruits and vegetables are good and should be thought of in a different category than the carbohydrates from grains and starches like breads, pasta, and potatoes. I view this as a problem with the way we classify carbohydrates more than anything else. Our knowledge base just hasn't expanded enough to separate these into two different categories of carbohydrates yet.

The other way to protect your muscle mass and not lose it while you are on any kind of weight loss journey is to exercise. Most patients think of running, jogging, or walking when I tell them about exercise. Those cardio forms of exercise are vitally important and help to keep your heart in good condition. But they are more for long-term health. When you are losing weight, you need to do muscle resistance exercises. Generally, this involves the use of weights, but you can utilize body weight exercises as a sole method if you prefer that instead. Utilizing the muscles you have will encourage your body to make good use of the protein you are consuming in your diet. I'm also not suggesting that you need to bulk up like a bodybuilder. Most people could benefit from gaining some muscle but even maintaining the muscle mass you already have is a victory when you are losing weight either on your own or with the help of GLP-1 medications. It is vitally important that you maintain your muscle mass for your long-term quality of life.

I hope this illustrates just how important dietary changes and exercise are for any weight loss journey. There is no substitute for either one of those. GLP-1 medications can make this process easier, but if you want to have sustained weight loss, you must commit to lifestyle changes. However, with the medication, you see the results of these changes so much quicker than trying to lose weight without the medication. We tend to struggle with delayed gratification and instead we want instant feedback in every aspect of our lives. This is especially true if we are doing something hard like weight loss. I believe that is a key reason we are in the midst of an obesity epidemic. Most of us have tried to lose weight before for a short time—a week, two weeks, a month, two months. And what happens when we make those hard changes and commit to a better, healthier lifestyle? We either don't lose any weight or the number on the scale goes up. That provides a huge amount of discouragement, and most of us give up when that happens. The reason this happens is because per square inch, muscle mass weighs more than body fat does. So, if you start losing body fat and gaining muscle mass, your total body weight goes up. Once again, we are seeing how our bodies work and produce a result that discourages us from losing weight. Therefore, it is no surprise that the majority of diets fail, leaving most adults overweight or obese.

Utilizing Advances with GIP to Fight Addictions

Another reason why we struggle with weight loss so much is that food addictions are a real thing even if we don't recognize them. Although I fully believe there are true food addictions, I also would lump emotional eating into this category. Emotional eating is when you consume food because you are happy, because you are sad, because you are worried or stressed, . . . or even just because food is available. Those cupcakes look good . . . or that cake smells good, so you have some even though you are not hungry at all.

A food addiction may involve a lack of willpower, but it may also involve using food as a reward. After a long, difficult meeting, you eat a cookie. Or you have a snack for the ride home after work because, "Gosh darn it, I deserve it!" All these forms of calorie intake result in a dopamine release in the brain. Dopamine is the reward chemical in our brains. Whenever you feel good after accomplishing something, you get that release of dopamine in the brain. Dopamine is also what triggers a lot of addictions—both illegal drug addictions and more harmless addictions. Our brains love dopamine and will work to get you to do things that result in a dopamine release. Remember my first day on the medication when I couldn't eat ice cream with my family? In the past, I would not have admitted that I was an emotional eater, but certainly I was. Ice cream released dopamine in my brain and caused me to want that dopamine release more and more.

The newest GLP-1 medication to the market, Mounjaro or Zepbound, have the active medication called tirzepatide and a newly discovered hormone in them that works in the brain to help people who struggle with these addictions and eating habits. It is called Glucose-dependent Insulinotropic Polypeptide (GIP) and certainly sets Mounjaro and Zepbound apart from the other medications in this class. None of the other GLP-1 medications (e.g., Ozempic, Wegovy) have this dual action component.

I believe that it was the GIP component that helped me break my own addiction to soda that I had struggled with for decades and never really had success with stopping prior to taking the medication. In addition to suppressing the appetite and promoting a prolonged feeling of fullness, Mounjaro and Zepbound also break that food-reward cycle and can enable people to break their food addiction problems because of the GIP component. It takes away the emotional component of food consumption and allows us to view our diet with a new unclouded lens where we can really evaluate why we are eating.

What gets really interesting is that, just as I was able to overcome my ice cream reward eating and soda addiction, some of my patients stopped drinking alcohol as a result of this medication. And some overcame other addictions while on these medications. And once again I'm left thinking that these medications are just too good to be true.

KEY POINTS

- ☛ Weight loss is unnatural.
- ☛ Plateaus will occur.
  - ‣ The weight loss journey is more of a step-down process than a curve.
  - ‣ GLP-1 medications make breaking through plateaus much easier.
- ☛ The old food pyramid was upside down.
  - ‣ Protein is good, and we tend to not get enough.
- ☛ Exercise is needed to maintain muscle mass.
- ☛ Addictions and emotional eating are the result of dopamine release in the brain.
  - ‣ Dopamine is the reward hormone.
  - ‣ The newest GLP-1 medication, Mounjaro and Zepbound, has a component that stops dopamine release in the brain from food intake.

Chapter 7

REST – HOW SLEEP AND STRESS FACTOR INTO WEIGHT LOSS

Sometimes, you are doing everything right and just not getting the results you want (or deserve). When that happens to me, my natural tendency is to just work harder until I finally achieve the desired results. It took me a long time to realize that sometimes pushing harder just isn't the best path forward. As hard as it was for me to embrace, resting and sleeping are important parts of the weight loss journey. Rest is so important that I would argue it is a nonnegotiable for success in your weight loss journey. Without good quality sleep, weight loss is just not possible. Stress is also a critical factor, so we will discuss both these issues in this chapter.

Rest Is Essential

We have all heard that sleep is vital for healthy living. Sleep is when our bodies do all those things that we never really think about. That includes things like healing, processing stress, recovering physically and emotionally from the day, and even fostering your dreams about the future (whoever told you dreams are pointless was lying!). Trying to lose weight without getting good quality sleep is just pointless.

Although we factor many things into preparing for the weight loss journey, few people prioritize sleep as an essential for weight loss. Sleep is just too easy to push off when you need to get one more thing accomplished before bedtime. It's also easy for early risers to shave thirty to sixty minutes off their sleep schedule in the morning to accomplish more in the day. That is where I always find "extra" time to get more things done! My favorite drug, caffeine, makes this incredibly easy . . . or at least more manageable. Shortchanging sleep, though, ends up harming us in the long run and ruins our chances of accomplishing our weight loss goal.

Whatever you are trying to accomplish by cutting into your sleep time is important, I'm sure. I always believed that. Let's not even consider that you are bingeing on your favorite show's new season on Netflix (or for the younger readers, bingeing on mindlessly scrolling through social media). Let's pretend that you are sacrificing sleep for something that is actually important and offers the chance to be more productive in life. I'm not trying to argue that you shouldn't do what you need to get done or that you should never sacrifice sleep for an important task. But I am trying to create the mindset that you need to make sleep just as much of a priority as whatever you are trying to get done at the expense of sleep.

Cutting into your sleep time may offer short-term rewards. Perhaps you can do a little extra research for your presentation or put the finishing touches on the project that has a rapidly approaching deadline. But was sleep the only thing that you could cut to accomplish that result? After all, you are trying to lose weight, so wouldn't it have been better to cut out the time it took to eat a snack instead?

Allowing your body to get enough sleep—good quality sleep—will greatly benefit you over time. When your body isn't getting the sleep that it needs, it goes into a stress response, and that response causes your body to go into a survival mode where you will hold onto weight a lot harder than you normally would. Survival mode scrapes for every extra calorie it can get in your diet and doesn't make the weight loss process easier. The problem is, most Americans don't know what being out of survival mode is even like. We live most of our working years, especially if you have young children, in this mode and then simply mask the effects of sleep deprivation with caffeine. That helps us get by day to day in the short term but doesn't help our long-term health at all. In this chapter, I don't discuss the long-term health risks associated with sleep deprivation, which are well-documented; instead, I will focus on how sleep deprivation negatively affects your weight loss goals.

Not All Sleep Is Equal

I tell patients that it is impossible to lose weight without good quality sleep. That's brash, but it gets the point across. I also stress the word *quality* associated with sleep in this discussion. That's because there is a night-and-day difference between lying in your bed, unconscious with your eyes closed for eight hours and lying in your bed cycling through the normal sleep stages. Just the act of resting or lying down with your eyes closed doesn't accomplish a whole lot. We intuitively know that this is true if we think about it. The most common experience with this kind of "rest" for most people is the sleep you get after a night of drinking alcohol. You might get eight hours of sleep (resting with eyes closed), but you don't wake up feeling refreshed. Even without having a hangover the next morning, you still don't feel fantastic. That's because alcohol stops your brain and body from cycling through the normal sleep stages. Without that normal cycling of the sleep stages, you aren't getting refreshed, and your body isn't getting the full benefits of sleep. It's not good *quality* sleep.

If you struggle to believe this, try one of the devices that track your sleep. There's a range of devices to choose from—apps, rings, watches, phones—that can tell you about your patterns as you cycle through the sleep stages. Although some of these devices aren't super accurate about what they are tracking, they do demonstrate that your body is cycling through different phases as you sleep. So, we don't want to use this data to make healthcare decisions, but it can show you whether you are cycling through some sleep stages or not. When you drink alcohol, you don't cycle through those phases, and it is detrimental to how you feel the next day. Your body becomes physically stressed by a lack of good quality sleep even though you are lying in bed with your eyes closed for several hours. So, the lack of quality rest pushes you further into survival mode, and it makes weight loss even harder to achieve.

Stress Has Real Consequences

Stress, especially emotional stress, can do this as well. Stress is a very real thing; it's not just in our heads. It has real, wide-ranging physical consequences in the human body, and most of those consequences are detrimental to us. I'm sure you have had a horrible night's sleep when you were wrestling with a big life decision, and as a result, your brain and body just didn't get the needed rest. The following day, you are foggy and not able to function well. We all experience emotional stress. Everyone encounters stress in their day-to-day life—even those people who don't admit it. Some people can respond to emotional stress very well, and others seem to get tripped up by it. But their response to the actual stress itself isn't even what I'm talking about. I'm more focused on how they process the stress they encounter rather than how they respond to that stressor. The big difference between those two is that some people are able to channel their stress into some stress-relieving activity that helps them process it and get rid of it.

Medicine doesn't have a great way to conceptualize or explain this concept. Sometimes, though, it is better to just give up on the task at hand for a bit and take a break to de-stress in order to keep things moving in the right direction. This is especially true for weight loss. Managing your stress and having a dedicated system to process the stress is vitally important. To do this, you must get to know yourself and be able to recognize when you are becoming stressed out. Then, develop the fortitude to stop the task at hand and switch to your stress management process or routine. For some people, this process looks like taking a break and watching a movie; for others it's going outside and exercising or calling a friend to chat. It doesn't matter what your stress management process is, but it vitally matters that you have one and can recognize when to use it so that you don't hold onto stress.

Yes, this may mean that you need to be less productive in the short term, but the long-term payoff is worth it. Most importantly, do what de-stresses you the most effectively; of course, the specific activity will vary from one person to another. I would much rather see a patient sit on the couch for thirty minutes zoning out and doing nothing as a way of de-stressing rather than have them push through the stress to hit a project deadline or force themselves to do some physical activity instead of processing their stress. In this example the act of exercising could create more stress and make the whole problem worse.

The key here is to learn what works best as a de-stressor for you, and even that may vary depending upon the situation you are facing. Everyone is so different in what de-stresses them. Whether it is watching TV, doing yoga, going for a run, chatting with a friend on the phone, or cleaning, it doesn't matter. The important thing is to find something that helps you process the stress you are feeling instead of internalizing it or holding onto it indefinitely. It also means that sometimes if you are stressed and you are not getting enough good quality sleep, you might need to skip the morning workout and get an extra hour of sleep instead to help you break through a plateau on your weight loss journey.

Remember that we are trying to make those big lifestyle changes that will result in long-term weight loss. The only way to accomplish big lifestyle changes is to make them sustainable for the long term. And getting only five or six hours of sleep night after night is not sustainable for most people, nor is it sustainable to live in a constant high stress state for months on end. Quality of life matters, and it matters a lot, so you must factor that into the decisions you make day to day on your weight loss journey.

Prioritizing Your Daily Values

For me, getting the rest I needed meant that I had to put my morning runs on pause for a while. I was one of those people who truly enjoyed running. I would intentionally wake up early to go for a run . . . and even crazier, I would run outside as long as it was warmer than ten degrees! I enjoyed being outdoors, even though it was in the middle of our town. I enjoyed seeing our streets empty and feeling like I had the whole neighborhood to myself. This was useful time for me as well. In addition to getting some physical activity in, I used this time to think about my day, plan out conversations I needed to have, listen to a news podcast so I was up to date with current events, and make sure I was maximizing my schedule for the day as much as possible. Not only was this incredibly useful time for me, but it was also physical activity that was helping me burn calories. I told myself that I could not function as productively or at as high of a level as I was currently functioning without my morning run.

However, on my weight loss journey, I came to the realization that my morning routine of running at the expense of an extra hour of sleep was more harmful than it was beneficial. This was a shocking realization that I did not like at all. I did not want it to be true. But the benefits of this physical activity didn't outweigh the negatives caused by the lack of sleep I was accumulating day after day. I was trying to lose weight and from an outsider's perspective, I was doing all the right things. However, I was still struggling and not seeing the number on the scale get lower despite my best efforts.

Once I gave up on this morning routine and gave sleep the priority it deserved, I found myself feeling better. I didn't rely on caffeine so much throughout the day. I still needed it (used it for sure!), but it was an "add on," not a requirement to keep the day moving. I found other times in my day to create my strategy or outline for the day in my head and listen to those podcasts—time that I oddly enough had not seen previously as an option to accomplish those tasks. My morning commute to work became that time for me. Instead of listening to a podcast for fun or listening to Spotify music, my commute provided a window of opportunity for accomplishing those tasks.

This example illustrates that we likely have tremendous blind spots in our lives. You read that last paragraph and probably thought, "duh . . . doing those things on your mindless commute to work was an obvious solution" but to me, in the moment and sleep-deprived, that thought had never even crossed my mind. We can't judge or even help each other out with this process. This is something that requires a lot of motivation to reprioritize things in your life after you do your own introspection and self-assessment. After all, you have lived several decades of your life and that cumulative experience has made you do things the way that you are doing them. If there was a better way to do them, you probably would have switched to that better way already. Therefore, you must reprioritize your daily values and then work forward from that reprioritized list of things that need to get accomplished each day. And when you reprioritize your daily values, getting good quality sleep and having a stress processing system must be high on that list. Even if that means giving up things you think you can't live without right now.

Don't reevaluate everything all in one sitting or as a spur of the moment exercise. Instead, take your time and think about this. Write your daily priorities down on paper, make this an in-depth exercise that will actually result in a change in your life and daily routine. Remember that quality of life is very important, and you are trying to make long-lasting lifestyle changes that you can sustain for years (or decades). You are on a weight loss journey. This journey never ends; therefore, it is important that these changes are sustainable in the long term.

KEY POINTS

- ☞ Good quality sleep is vitally important for weight loss.
  - ➤ There is a huge difference between total sleep time and quality sleep time.
- ☞ Stress management is needed for weight loss.
  - ➤ We all have stress.
  - ➤ You must process your stress so the body can lose weight.
- ☞ Determine your daily priorities and values.
  - ➤ Examine your routines and fine-tune them.

Chapter 8

TRACKING DATA AND BUILDING RELATIONSHIPS

We are creatures of routine who thrive in relationships, so build systems that hijack those routines and maximize your relationships.

Tracking the Right Data

We are in the age of data. There is so much new data all around us. We can wear devices that track not only our location but also our vital signs on a minute-by-minute basis. In the previous chapter, I mentioned that apps, rings, watches, and phones can be used to track different phases of sleep. It's an unbelievable time to be alive! In fact, when my patients get excited about some new device that offers to track some aspect of their health, I often have more fear than excitement about it. That's because most things about our bodies that are easy to track don't really offer that much insight into our overall health. The main goal that I have for my patients is to help them live not just a long life, but to have a great quality of life for as long as possible. Therefore, knowing that their respiration rate is 18 for two hours every afternoon doesn't really help me (or them) accomplish their main goal all that much. In fact, it is often more detrimental than positive because it gives them something to stress about if they are not in the "normal" category (the normal category that a computer engineer decided, which might not be relevant to any human activity). Ugh!

However, it is also widely known that you can't improve things that you don't track. The only way to improve something is to be aware of it and have a way to measure it. Therefore, you must track the things that you want to improve over time if you want to change that behavior. Weight is an obvious data point to track when you are trying to lose weight. Most smartphones have an app in which you can enter a daily weight (or weekly weight) and have the app graph the data out for you so you can see your progress at a glance. The app can even create trends for you and alert you if your trend is moving in the wrong direction. For things that you want to change—and have a process in place to change—this kind of tracking is a fantastic tool to use.

In the previous paragraph, I mentioned that you could use a device to track daily weight or weekly weight. Let's pause here for a moment and use this as an opportunity to address the matter of adaptability and personalization. I tell my patients not to track daily weights but to track weekly or monthly weight instead . . . or not even to weigh themselves at all but to go by how their clothes are fitting and how they feel day to day. That's mainly because too many factors can influence weight at any one point in time. For instance, water is incredibly heavy relative to most other things in the body. When you wake up and realize you gained two pounds from the previous day despite doing everything right, it can be very discouraging. If you are just more hydrated at the time and that two pounds isn't "real" even though it shows up on the scale, you have gained bad data that isn't helpful at all. That bad data will mess up your graphs and trends while also providing bad feedback on your progress. Getting down into the weeds with how much fluid you consume day to day or how much salt or protein or how much you used your muscles the day before is too much for patients to track and process. Therefore, it's easier to space out the data collection points of their weight to weekly or monthly to avoid getting disappointed even when they know they are doing the right things. You are much more likely to capture a helpful data point and trend by spacing out the collection points.

With that said, I track my weight daily, and it's not because I'm tracking all those variables. Instead, I weigh myself daily because it helps my mental health and lessens my anxiety to have a specific data point each day. I don't put any weight (pun intended!) or value in any one data point on my weight because I am aware of those variables. Instead, I just enter the data into my phone and then let the app create a trend for me over time. This approach has worked best for me, but it doesn't work for a lot of patients. Therefore, you must know yourself well enough to get the data you need in the least stressful way. Adapt to how you are tracking things but keep the overall goal in mind. Finding a way to be ruthlessly practical with these routines and data collection points is the key to success.

Besides weight, tracking what you eat is incredibly valuable. I'm not talking about anything sophisticated like how much carbs versus proteins you are taking in each day. Instead, just writing down what you put in your mouth each day is eye-opening for a lot of people. It is so easy to forget about those worthless calories you consumed as you ran out the door or the small bite of dessert that you tried even though you felt like you were being "good" and containing yourself. But once you commit to writing down everything that goes in your mouth, you will likely realize that you are consuming a lot of things throughout the day. Furthermore, most Americans are consuming a lot more than anyone needs to survive. I'm not trying to be a downer here, and you still need to enjoy life, but just about every American could cut back on the volume of food they consume daily. Cutting back on the volume will help decrease the size of your stomach, which provides additional benefits that I have discussed elsewhere in this book.

Tracking Puts You in Control

The point of tracking a couple of data points is to help you effect change in your lifestyle. Our current reality is a result of what we tolerate and allow into our lives. Whether we think about it or not, we all have learned to deal with or tolerate some things while actively avoiding others. The systems and processes we have developed that automatically make these decisions for us lead us to our current reality (i.e., what we allow in our lives and our current situation). Whether we know it or not, we have designed these systems that interact with the world in such a way as to provide the results we are getting for ourselves. This is mind-blowing the first time you fully comprehend it and realize the impact it has on your life in general. Everything we do affects, maybe even determines, how we are living each day. Knowing this can feel overwhelming . . . or at least it did for me.

However, after you get over that initial shock, you realize that this means you can change those systems and thereby change your current reality. You are in charge, so only you can make those changes. That's good news too because the only person you can control is yourself. Therefore, to change those systems, you must first track the results and then experiment with ways to change those results. The difficulty is that we are experts at deceiving ourselves; we are also the first to believe our foolish excuses. It is so much easier to lie to yourself than anyone else. That's why a food diary (tracking your food consumption) or tracking your weight can be a valuable aid. They help you see what is working and what isn't working. Because right now, I guarantee that whatever you are doing is producing the results that you are currently experiencing. To make a change, you require objective data to stop lying to yourself and take the hard steps of changing your daily routines and activities.

Building Beneficial Relationships

Relationships function in much the same way; that is, you can tolerate some people and avoid others. What you choose to tolerate and avoid determines who you allow into your life. We maintain relationships that we created for better or for worse. For instance, you might not like your boss, but you tolerate the relationship to get a paycheck every week. Sure, it might seem impossible to change jobs right now, but you know that the only way to change that relationship is for you to get a better boss. But you may decide that it isn't worth the risk and hassle to make that change in your life right now. Therefore, you tolerate the relationship because you think that making the change would cost more than its worth. That's just a flawed example of what I'm trying to illustrate here, but the fact is we have much more control over our day-to-day lives than we allow ourselves to realize. Relationships fall squarely into this category. We are so good at lying to ourselves, giving ourselves the benefit of the doubt, and manipulating our own emotions that we fail to see what might be possible. This is all subconscious, of course, so it does require work to take off those blinders and realize the truth all around you.

So, you must evaluate whether your relationships with others are worthwhile and beneficial. Please don't think that I'm arguing that you should only be in relationships that are beneficial to you. Taking care of your kids isn't a financially beneficial relationship, but it certainly is worthwhile . . . and we would all agree on that. But do you have relationships that are stopping your forward progress on your weight loss journey? Do you go out to lunch with a coworker who overeats even though that makes it harder for you to not overeat? Or what about your friend who constantly makes bad food choices and puts you in situations (or restaurants) where there aren't any great choices that help your weight loss journey. Sometimes, it's beneficial to reevaluate those relationships, whatever that looks like. Reevaluating relationships can be challenging, which is why most of us fail at making the big changes that would result in significant progress toward our goals. It's also why most of us have failed to sustain previous weight loss over the years. We have not fully committed to lifelong lifestyle changes because they are so hard and disruptive to our comfortable lives.

That might seem harsh at first, but it doesn't have to be. You can choose to go for a walk with that coworker instead of going out to lunch or do something active with your friend instead of getting appetizers and drinks together. You have to change something if you want different results. Utilize your relationships to help you achieve your goals. Because if you don't, you will be stuck in the process and routines that you have created—the same ones that have made the situation you are currently in.

My Practical Example

For me, that looked like changing the way I consumed food at work. Previously, I would get take-out with coworkers three to five times each week. It was fun, and it was social. It made me feel good and allowed a break from the stressors of the office. It certainly released dopamine in my brain. However, because I was tracking my food intake, I knew it was a vulnerable time for me when I would overeat and consume too many calories. I first tried to eat less or eat only half of whatever portion I would get. However, I proved to myself time and again that I did not have the willpower to stop eating and do that. I tried only ordering healthy options, but honestly a lot of healthy fast-food options are bad options.

I had to make the hard decision to stop eating with coworkers all together. I did not like making this decision, but I was in a bad place with my health, and I had to take drastic action to change it. I had to stop blaming others and stop accepting the lies I was telling myself. The change wasn't easy for me, but it proved to be even harder when coworkers started reacting negatively about this change. Some thought that I had developed an eating disorder because they didn't see me overeating all the time. For me, this change was worth the cost. I was on a mission to lose weight, and I knew that I had to change the routines and processes or systems that were causing me to be overweight. Especially now that I'm on the other side of my weight loss journey and have systems and processes in place to help keep me in a good routine, it seems so obvious. I wish I had realized the need to change much sooner.

I'm still friends with my coworkers; nothing has changed between us except I don't eat lunch with them anymore. The horrible outcomes that I feared would happen if I stopped eating lunch with them never came true. I still talk with them and interact throughout the day, so my fear that I wouldn't be accepted by them was completely unfounded. That was just a lie I had created and believed for years in order to keep doing the same thing—mainly overeating and getting that dopamine release in my brain. With those blinders on though, it's very hard to imagine what a different reality can look like or how to change things to get to that new reality. That's why you must have objective data that doesn't lie to you so you can figure out how to get better results by changing your daily routines, systems, processes, and relationships. The double-edged sword is that only *you* can make these vital changes.

KEY POINTS

- ☛ You are exactly where you have allowed yourself to be.
  - ➤ Your routines and systems have allowed you to become who you are.
  - ➤ Lifestyle changes are needed for weight loss.
- ☛ The only way to know that you changed something is to track it.
  - ➤ Improvement will only come after you analyze your situation and make a change.
- ☛ Relationships help to make lifestyle changes easier and longer lasting.

Chapter 9

MAINTENANCE – WEANING OFF MEDICATION AND KEEPING THE WEIGHT OFF

A s we previously discussed, weight loss is unnatural. Over thousands of years, humans lived in situations where there was a scarcity of food, and they alternated between feast and famine. Thus, holding onto extra calories became an evolutionary advantage because you could never be sure where your next meal would be coming from or even what your next meal would consist of. Contrast that with our society where food is abundant and readily accessible. We plan our meals out in advance and know exactly where our next meal will come from . . . and even what it will be. If you don't partake of the food in some situations, you are considered rude . . . a birthday cake at a birthday party or a new food that a friend or loved one has spent hours making. For most of us, calories are readily available and abundant.

We are living in unprecedented times where there is an abundance of food and most of us know how to easily get more food. That is so different from any other point in human history. We can even use DoorDash or UberEats to get virtually any kind of food we want quickly. Historically, humans had to search for food and then work to prepare it. We live in an environment where we can consume significantly more calories while also working less to obtain those calories. The natural result of those forces is that we gain weight year after year.

Fad Diets Are Bad

Trying a fad diet here and there might have helped you lose weight for a short time, but it didn't last. The weight came back and probably brought some extra weight with it, so you ended up weighing more than when you started the fad diet. That gets to the heart of why I hate fad diets . . . because they all have an end date. After that end date, you go back to your normal diet and rhythms that caused you to gain weight in the first place, so of course, the weight doesn't stay off. That's because you didn't change anything in your life.

Therefore, to lose weight **and** keep the weight off, the changes you make have to become a new lifestyle for you. As I shared earlier, you have to imagine that these GLP-1 medications are training wheels or guardrails that will help you stay on the correct path. But if you stop the medication, you must stay on that same path—just without the training wheels or guardrails. Easier said than done, I know. But is losing weight and gaining it back such a bad thing? I believe it certainly is bad to repeatedly lose the same ten pounds for some big event (like a wedding) and then gain it right back afterward. Yo-yoing is not something to be happy about or celebrated. Our bodies can adapt to a lot of things. Since weight loss is unnatural, once you trick your body into losing weight by a certain method, the second time you want to lose weight by that method, it will become much harder. The body doesn't want to be tricked again and will adapt and learn how to react to whatever fad you are using.

Lifestyle Changes Are Necessary

The fad diet trend highlights the importance of using GLP-1 medications to augment your own natural weight loss regimen and then committing to following that regimen even after you stop the medication. That is the only way to get sustained weight loss. It also demonstrates that we might only have one, two, or three chances with the medication when they will work so effectively. Nobody knows for sure, but it certainly is a fear that I have talked to all my patients about. Just because the medication worked so well for them now, I'm not 100 percent sure it will work just as well in a few years if the weight does come back. You **must** learn to change your lifestyle and habits to maintain weight loss.

Eating dramatically less when you go out to eat, late night snacking, and consuming mindless calories solely because food is available must become a thing of the past if you want to maintain the weight loss you achieved on the GLP-1 medication. If you aren't ready to make those big lifestyle changes, then the medication might do more harm than good in the long term. Yes, you would likely still lose weight the first time on the medication, but the weight is going to come back unless you make real changes to your lifestyle. And you will have wasted a weight loss chance with the medication that your body might never offer you again.

Weaning Off Gradually

Part of how I encourage patients to maintain weight loss is in the way I wean them off the medication. I don't think it is right to yank away the medication after they hit their goal. That would be like saying, "Wow, you did great and accomplished your goal; now go back to your normal life and the habits that made you overweight in the first place." That's just not a good message or path forward for patients. To help patients maintain their successful weight loss, I set up loose guardrails and training wheels for them. Once both the patient and I are happy with their weight and it's a healthy weight to maintain, we switch to a maintenance mode to wean off the medication. Instead of doing one injection every week, I first push them out to one injection every two weeks. This allows them to feel what life is like without the medication in their system. They can feel unrestricted hunger again and their full feeling won't be amplified either. They are taking off the training wheels for a week, but they know that they can put them right back on the following week. Patients are bound to make some missteps, and it's exceedingly helpful for them to know they have the comfort of the medication to fall back on.

Once they can maintain their new weight steadily for two weeks at a time, we space the medication out to three weeks with the same thought pattern. They can be without the training wheels of the medication for two weeks and then rely on the medication for a week. After the three-week frequency, they switch to once-a-month dosing. For the most part this is an easy transition from the three-week dosing because by then, they have established the proper guardrails themselves without the medication to keep the weight off. They know what their triggers are and can avoid them, or they have a system in place to help them say no to them.

After using the medication for one week each month, we then discuss stopping the medication all together. This is the hardest step for most patients because they have likely developed an emotional connection with the medication itself. For the first time in their lives, they were able to achieve the long-desired goal of drastic weight loss. The emotional attachment to the medication makes it hard for them to say goodbye to it so quickly. Plus, they have seen what happened when they stopped previous weight loss attempts only to have had all their weight return (and then some). Therefore, most of my patients opt to stay on once-a-month dosing for a longer period than I think is necessary. However, I let them do so for their mental health, the confidence boost, and continued education in how to handle certain situations (e.g., holidays, vacations, parties). After a year at their lower weight though, I make a concerted effort to have them stop the medication completely. Their metabolic set point should have "reset" by this point, and it should be easier for them to maintain the new lower weight.

Maintaining your new lower weight while weaning off the medication takes work. I often tell patients to turn the food pyramid that they grew up with upside down. Focus on getting enough protein (actual amounts vary from person to person) because protein is filling but also helps maintain the weight loss. Increased protein is especially needed along with muscle resistance exercises to avoid losing muscle mass while on the medications. I also stress the importance of getting good quality sleep. Sure, you might be able to function on four or five hours of sleep, but your metabolism isn't going to like that. Stress is a very real thing; it has real-world consequences that can result in weight gain. Sleep helps you process that stress, so good quality sleep is vital for losing weight and maintaining weight loss.

I also have a discussion with patients about what weight they want to maintain after weight loss. Everyone has a different idea about this. Some are completely comfortable gaining back five of the pounds they lost if that means they can have more desserts with their family. Others find comfort in their new healthier lifestyle and want to keep off every pound. Factoring their wishes into our decision about the medication is vital. No one wants to live to be 100 if you can't do anything you enjoy. What are they comfortable maintaining? Life is meant for living, so constantly depriving yourself can lead to bad feelings and ultimately make the weight come back. Finding moderation is key to everything. Then working with the patient to hold them accountable for maintaining that moderation is equally as valuable.

KEY POINTS

- ☛ There are evolutionary advantages to holding onto extra weight.

- ☛ Weight loss is hard and unnatural.

- ☛ Most people have had bad experiences with fad diets.

  - › Fad diets can do more harm than good.

- ☛ GLP-1 medications work best as guardrails or training wheels to make lifestyle changes.

  - › They make it easier to sustain those lifestyle changes.

  - › Lifestyle changes are what really matter with weight loss.

- ☛ Weaning off the medication can be challenging.

  - › Use a thoughtful approach to stopping the medication.

  - › Spacing out injections has advantages.

  - › To reset your set point, you must maintain weight loss for a while.

- ☛ Develop an individualized plan to maintain weight loss.

  - › Factor quality of life into that plan.

  - › Moderation is key for everything.

Chapter 10

THE FUTURE OF MEDICINE

Now that I have sustained success with weight loss using GLP-1 medications and the strategies we discussed, it's tough for me not to get excited when thinking about what the future holds. I am an eternal optimist at heart, and that factors into how I view the future of medicine and specifically these medications. Whether I need to go back on the medication for a couple months every few years, get into a more regular maintenance regimen, or maybe never even use them again, I view these medications as a great thing despite their side effects and all the unknowns that come with them.

The benefits of losing weight have been well-documented over the last fifty years and provide the foundation for most of our current practice of medicine. After all, excessive weight contributes to most of the health issues I treat day in and day out. High blood pressure, type 2 diabetes, high cholesterol, fatty liver disease, arthritis, and sleep apnea have a component of weight related to them. Losing weight would greatly improve these conditions or maybe even eliminate them all together for certain individuals. That's what I was taught in medical school, and that is what every respected major medical organization acknowledges as well. I've seen success with my own patients . . . their blood pressure improves, their sleep apnea goes away, they feel better, and their joints no longer ache. It's a game changer for primary care, and this is the first time in my career that I have seen these issues improve or go away. The medical community knows that one of the biggest issues in medicine right now is the excessive weight we carry around.

Abundant Opportunities for Improvement

In addition to the immediate benefits of weight loss, there are many long-term effects of having patients lose weight to completely eliminate their high blood pressure or diabetes. The potential to dramatically reduce the number of heart attacks and strokes over the next ten to twenty years becomes even more exciting to think about. We could potentially have a solution for most of our society's current medical issues. But to make the medications more broadly available, insurance companies would have to cover the cost of the medication. Right now, most insurance companies don't view obesity as a true medical condition; instead, they view it as a lifestyle issue and therefore they don't cover medications used to treat weight loss. That's crazy and ridiculous, especially when you think about how much money we would save the healthcare system by helping individuals with this aspect of their lives. That doesn't even consider the individual benefits that patients would get from losing weight. But insurance companies know that most people switch insurance coverage every three years. Therefore, they are very short-sighted when they make their decisions. If they paid for these expensive medications, they would only be saving money for one of their competitors since it would prevent health issues from occurring years down the road.

My proposal for this problem is to have the major medical organizations that develop our treatment guidelines or algorithms work these new medications into the treatment of various health conditions. These treatment guidelines and algorithms dictate what insurance companies must cover. If there is a proven benefit to taking a medication for a health condition and it's the only medication available for that condition, they would have to cover it. Imagine an individual in their mid- to late-forties who comes to see me. Their blood pressure is borderline, their cholesterol is borderline, and their blood sugar is borderline . . . all on top of being forty pounds overweight. This is a common scenario that I see and treat frequently, usually with pharmaceutical medications. Each of these medical conditions requires a pharmaceutical medication after the patient fails to make the lifestyle changes that we always recommend and try first. Therefore, the patient ends up on multiple medications that control their problems, but they don't get to the root cause of the issue or reverse anything. We are only managing their issues. What if, instead of starting three medications, we did a trial of the GLP-1 medication for a few months? Then the patient has a much higher likelihood of losing weight and making sustained lifestyle changes. This success can motivate them to pursue other areas of improvement for their health like the ones we discussed earlier. Typically, one win leads to wins in other aspects of their lives. Getting the major guideline organizations to incorporate the use of these medications at an early stage would force insurance companies to cover the medications. The result would be a much healthier population and the real possibility of changing the course of health for our society.

If this could be accomplished, our society would have the chance to prevent most causes of high blood pressure, high cholesterol, and diabetes—not all of them, but the incidence of these three would go down drastically. We also know that these three conditions are the major cause of heart attacks and strokes years down the road. Therefore, preventing these conditions or even just delaying them by ten years or so would have major positive implications for our society. And at the individual level, it would result in more years with a better quality of life. If you are going to live longer, you need to have a good quality of life.

Just As Impactful As Antibiotics

To help illustrate the potential impact I see that these medications can have on our society, I often compare them to the introduction of antibiotics into the practice of medicine. Prior to antibiotics, patients would die or get severe complications from simple bacterial infections such as skin infections and pneumonias. Everyone who got an infection was at risk, not just elderly or immunocompromised individuals. All that changed in the early 1900s when antibiotics began to be mass-produced. With a simple pill, all those bad outcomes became much rarer (although occasionally they still do happen). Antibiotics freed our society from the grip of bacterial infections and offered a beautiful solution. With modern medicine, if an otherwise healthy person dies of a treatable bacterial infection, it would be considered a huge failure. We would be shocked. No one would blame the individual or say that their illness was a lifestyle choice because they worked in a way that predisposed them to infections.

This isn't to minimize all the side effects or bad things that can come from antibiotics such as antibiotic resistance. But we would agree that we live in a better world because antibiotics are readily available. The GLP-1 class of medications has the potential to make the same impact on our society and world. If we incorporate them into guidelines to reverse the root cause of heart attacks and strokes, we could change the trajectory of the people's health across the world. It would free up researchers and doctors to work on other things, which hold a lot of potential and promise.

The Mental Health Aspect

Finally, I need to touch on the mental health aspect of these medications that I alluded to earlier. In addition to an obesity epidemic in our society, we also have a mental health crisis. Rates of depression and anxiety have sky-rocketed in the last decade. Doctors don't understand the reason for this trend, and I am sure there are multiple contributing factors. I was astonished at the improvement in my own mental health after I lost weight. Although I wasn't depressed or anxious at the outset of my weight loss journey, I definitely noticed an improvement in my mental condition after losing a significant amount of weight. The improvement in each of my patients who lost a significant amount of weight has been equally amazing. I love talking to those patients now because they are so full of hope and joy, and they have a positive outlook on life. These weren't deeply depressed or anxious individuals to begin with, just average people like you and me. But the weight loss resulted in a dramatic improvement in how they viewed their health and the world in general; it literally changed what they thought they were capable of doing in other aspects of their lives. Undoubtedly, helping people take a step in the right direction with their mental health is nothing but good. Empowering them to take control of their lives and produce lifestyle changes holds tremendous value for the patient but also for our greater society.

Weight loss is very complicated and our approach to helping patients with it is changing. These GLP-1 medications aren't for everyone, and I'm sure they won't work for everyone either. However, a large segment of our population could benefit greatly from the use of these medications. These medications facilitate improvements in those individuals' lives and the lives of their family members as well as society at large. That future is exciting to think about and one I want to live in. Practicing medicine in a world where I'm not always treating conditions that are brought on by our own excesses would be a game changer.

I'm not advocating that everyone should take these medications or even that everyone should lose weight. However, most adults in our society are overweight and struggle greatly to manage their weight, not to mention actually lose weight. They are on a slow path to a bad place, and I've seen it happen time and time again in patients that I care for. This new tool has the potential to help these individuals improve in a way that I would have thought impossible had I not tried it myself and witnessed these changes with my own eyes repeatedly. If you believe you are one of those individuals who could benefit from using medications, please reach out to your primary care doctor. Have a vulnerable conversation with them and talk about your previous failures with weight management and weight loss. Research your options and have an intelligent conversation with your primary care doctor. A lot of physicians are overworked and struggling with these same issues, so they might not be completely up to date with all the new medication options. But starting the conversation with a knowledgeable physician who knows the risks and benefits is a great place to begin to see how you can ultimately make needed lifestyle changes to provide sustained weight loss.

KEY POINTS

- ☛ Weight loss has proven and well-documented health benefits.

- ☛ Most of society's health problems stem from excessive weight.

- ☛ Widespread use of these medications would save the healthcare system lots of money.

- ☛ Adding GLP-1 medications to the guidelines for treating other weight-related illnesses holds the potential to get them covered by insurance companies.

- ☛ These medications are just as revolutionary as antibiotics were.

- ☛ Mental health improves with weight loss.

Chapter 11

IT'S NOT ONE THING . . .
IT'S EVERYTHING

Writing a book about weight or being a weight loss doctor was never my intention when I was in medical school. I was focused on practicing private direct primary care from the beginning of my career. That specialty area allowed me to really get to know my patients and struggle with them through their health care issues over the years. Going through that struggle with so many patients, I started to see patterns emerge. Weight was one of those patterns; every patient wanted to lose weight, and just about every patient failed to stop the upward trend of their weight over the years.

For better or worse, weight is an integral part of our identity; it literally affects everything we do and how we view ourselves. Changing your weight is often a slow painful process with minimal progress, which happens in small steps that are difficult to achieve. Patients are left wondering how much all that sacrifice of changing their weight really matters or changes their long-term health trajectory. Seeing patients struggle with losing weight repeatedly solidified just how important weight is to each and every one of us . . . and how it has its fingers in so many different aspects of our lives.

Losing weight fast allowed me to vividly recall what it was like before I lost weight. It didn't happen slowly over years the way I advised my patients to do before these GLP-1 medications became available. Instead, it took just a few short months for me to achieve a drastically lower weight. Therefore, I was able to look back, evaluate, and compare the stark differences.

Surprising Personal Benefits

For me, the change was dramatic and impactful. I felt better in general, I had more energy, I slept better, and my wife loved that I didn't snore anymore. I even noticed that I was thinking quicker and clearer than before, which was astonishing to me. My self-confidence improved, and I was able to take this win with the weight loss (that was made dramatically easier with the GLP-1 medications) and use that momentum to accomplish other goals that I had failed at achieving over the previous decade of my life. I was playing with my kids more after work and flirting more with my wife too. At work I wasn't so run down by five o'clock, so I could give my last patient of the day as much thought and clarity as I had for my first patient of the day. Suddenly, hard things didn't seem so hard to me. I had just accomplished this monumental task of losing the weight that I had wanted to lose for a whole decade. I felt like other difficult tasks wouldn't be so challenging after that. This new thought process and the changes that happened in me benefited not only myself but also the people around me—especially my family.

Mental health has never been given its rightful place in our society. I wouldn't say that I ever struggled with my mental health before, though I certainly had patients who struggled a lot more with it. I did know that mental health was a huge part of all our lives, but because of society's stigma, it often doesn't get addressed appropriately. The boost in mental health was so great for me that I couldn't help but talk to others about their own mental health. It's the lens through which we view reality, and I felt like I had found a new lens that was dramatically better. I wasn't so stressed about small things, my anxiety lessened, and of course my mood was better. Perhaps these changes were because I was getting better quality sleep because of the weight loss, but the cause didn't really matter to me. The improvement happened, I was enjoying it, and I wanted others to enjoy it as well.

Societal Benefits

Switching gears to think about the larger societal picture, just image what the possibilities might be if we "cured" our current obesity epidemic and at the same time had a wave of improvement in our country's mental health. Two of the biggest problems we are facing as a society would improve dramatically. Not only would it help individuals, but it would unlock the potential of thousands of individuals who are currently being held back by a mental health crisis that is exploding all around us. I've said it before, and I'll say it again; everyone needs hope on their horizon. They need something to look forward to and to be excited about. If these medications can help more people realize their full potential by making an unbelievably hard task suddenly more manageable so that they have the confidence to explore new options in their life, then we should be in favor of their use in our society.

Building off that, our health care system could be completely overhauled by the widespread use of these medications. A tremendous number of weight-related conditions plague our health care system. If we could reduce the amount of "wear and tear" arthritis on hips and knees, that would not only benefit the individual's quality of life in the short term, but it would benefit our health care system by reducing the number of joint replacement surgeries. Bariatric surgery that drastically alters your internal GI tract and physiology could become a relic of the past. That alone could save the healthcare system significantly and also improve the quality of life for many individuals. Certainly, carrying around less weight would lower cardiovascular risks, so it's possible that there would be significantly fewer heart attacks and strokes for the healthcare system to treat in the future. Fewer overweight and obese individuals would mean fewer diabetic patients and a reduction in the complications that come from diabetes. I often tell patients that I don't want any of them to become diabetic strictly because of how it dramatically decreases their quality of life.

It gets exciting to think about these changes at a broader level and how much less strained our healthcare system could be if we do have a cure or treatment for being overweight or obese. Just as antibiotics revolutionized medicine when they were discovered, these GLP-1 medications could usher in a new era of healthcare. It is equally exciting to think about the potential these changes might unlock in our healthcare system. Perhaps more time, energy, and resources would be focused on cancer or neurodegenerative disorders, which might lead to breakthroughs in those areas. There certainly would be a disruption in the current pharmaceutical industry as fewer people would need to take blood pressure, heart, and diabetic medications. Our screening process and utilization of testing in healthcare could change as well.

If patients feel better and have a better quality of life, that will also benefit our economy. More people would be willing to take vacations; they would have more time and energy to explore new hobbies and interests. They might even turn one of their hobbies into a business, which would benefit many people. The ripple effects are endless. It's all speculation right now, but it certainly is exciting to think about what the potential might be down the road.

After what I experienced, it's hard to not become excited about how these medications can impact so much for so many people. I am reminded by my success every day in various aspects of my life. Shaving my face has become harder now that I have more indentations in my neck instead of a fluffy smooth blob of skin. Crossing my legs when I sit is so much easier. I'm able to bend down and get up off the floor without a problem. My knees don't ache daily; instead, it now feels good to stand on one leg and bend down just because I can. My balance has improved. I am able to come home from work and pick my wife up to give her a kiss instead of just walking by her and saying hi. I've had all these changes, and I want others to have them as well. I've seen my patients have similar improvements, and I know it's not just something that uniquely happened to them or to me. It's possible to change your whole life, and it might start with one of the hardest things we have ever had to do . . . losing weight. But that task is dramatically easier now with these GLP-1 medications that hold the potential to change the world.

KEY POINTS

☛ Weight affects every aspect of our lives.

☛ The benefits of weight loss are wide-ranging, affecting multiple areas of our lives.

☛ Mental health improves with weight loss as well.

☛ The future is bright for society with GLP-1 medications.

AFTERWORD

I hope you enjoyed this book and that it motivated you to take the next step on whatever journey you are on. I've never seen a movement in medicine like this before, and I believe we are on the precipice of huge change in our society with these GLP-1 medications. One of the best ways to lose weight and keep weight off is to join a community of others who are doing the same thing that you are. That's why I created a weight loss coaching program that you can access to further understand how to best accomplish your weight loss goals, help motivate you to continue on the journey, wean off the medications, and maintain your weight loss goal.

The thing with weight loss is that there is never a destination; it's a process, a journey. Every meal, every opportunity for exercise, every chance to take the stairs or to park farther away is an opportunity for a healthier you. Choosing to do those actions every time can become an exhausting and overwhelming path to go down if you think you're alone. We all do better with encouragement and help from others, and I would love to see you succeed just as I have.

Go to my website www.DirectMDCoach.com to get connected and learn more. I can't wait to help you on this journey.

ABOUT THE AUTHOR

Jonathan Schmidt was born as the youngest of four boys to a father who was a mechanic and a stay-at-home mom. His oldest brother was the first in the family to go to college, and Jon was the first to get an advanced degree. He grew up loving baseball and basketball while also excelling in school. After suffering a broken arm at the age of three and being amazed at how the doctors could fix it, he started telling his mother that he wanted to be a doctor. That phrase continued to come out of his mouth as he got older. In his sophomore year of high school, he realized he needed to focus more on academics because his sports career wasn't going anywhere, and he got serious about becoming a doctor.

Jon graduated from his small high school in Illinois as salutatorian before attending Southern Illinois University in Carbondale. He majored in microbiology and earned a minor in chemistry. Once again, he excelled academically and graduated as one of the top 25 seniors in a class of almost 5,000 students. Next, he enrolled in medical school at the

University of Illinois where he read a book about concierge medicine and decided that was what he wanted to do with his career. He was accepted into a special alternative track for his third year of medical school called the Rural Student Physician Program where he got one-on-one experience from a small-town physician to hone his skills as a primary care doctor.

While in medical school, he married his wife, Cristal. They had met in high school but didn't start dating until college when they were 800 miles apart. They still joke that the distance is what enabled Jon to focus on academics instead of getting distracted with other things.

After medical school, Jon went to South Bend, Indiana, for Residency in Family Medicine. He continued to seek out concierge (or what is now called Direct Primary Care) opportunities and even designed a rotation specifically for himself at a thriving concierge clinic in Indianapolis. In his final year, he served as chief resident of the residency program.

That rotation led to his current job at one of the largest Direct Primary Care (DPC) practices in the nation. Due to the nature of DPC, he can focus on preventative healthcare with his patients and spend a good deal of time getting to know them on a personal level. Building relationships with his patients is one of the things that he enjoys most about how he practices medicine. These relationships are what led to his desire to improve health and the healthcare system by writing this book.

Jon enjoys spending time with his wife, Cristal, and their three children. When he isn't working, he likes to try new water sports on a local lake; he also enjoys woodworking and home DIY projects.

Milton Keynes UK
Ingram Content Group UK Ltd.
UKHW021119070624
443893UK00014B/765

9 781632 966759